VARiANT C-19

Robert Dresner

Library of Congress Control Number:
ISBN: 978-0-9854874-8-5

This book was printed in the United States of America, and published by Virga Press, LLC.

To order additional copies of this book, please contact:
Virga Press, LLC
P.O. Box 4881
Boulder, CO 80304
www.robertdresner.com
www.virgapress.com

For the love of life.

"If karma is the difference we perceive between ourselves and others, the painful and sinister gap between the *infected* and the healthy may never be breached."

Preface

I already wrote a few novels to good reviews, and never imagined I would write a non-fiction. But one of my doctors and several friends encouraged me write this book about the Covid-19 virus. They felt I needed to say these things in a way that is unique to myself, and that there are people who needed to hear them.

I hope they are right. The book is a creative journal, chronicling my experience with Covid-19, becoming sick in March 2020 and trying to heal amidst all the sadness and madness that has gripped our country throughout the pandemic.

As we all know, it has become impossible to separate the virus from politics, let alone myriad cultural issues, if only because the misuse of power has exacerbated the problem. Currently, there are more than 700,000 dead and 45 million infected in the U.S.

This virus is so strange and sinister, harming so many of us in so many ways, it may take a miracle to save us from ourselves, let alone the disease. And much more than the efforts of a new president. After all, we are in this together.

Robert

PS: Please know that much of this story is told in real time, when I was quite sick with the virus, long before I imagined it as a book; and that some elements have been juxtaposed to enhance the flow of the story. Also know that the text was lightly edited to preserve the rawness of my experience.

Other books by Robert Dresner

THE ASTRAL IMPERATIVE
Vol. I The Dream
Vol. II The Machine
Vol. III ReGenesis
Vol. IV Cosmos
Vol. V North Country

THE COMING
SATORI BLUES
THE KARMA CONSPIRACY

VARIANT

C-19

And so, it begins—weirdly.

1

It is sinister, this virus. Deadly. And it can be terribly painful in ways that are hard to imagine. They, the doctors, the scientists, the people telling us every day what they know—in effect telling us more about what they don't know, if only because so many people have already died. And you wonder if this madness will ever end despite the promise of the vaccines. Or maybe we simply save our precious selves with an injection of Lysol, as President Trump had suggested.

It was the evening of March 13 when the pain came; I went to sleep feeling pretty good at 10pm Woke up within a half-hour with creeping body pain in my joints, and then in my muscles, all over my body. Pain turned violent within an hour, dull nearest the skin, sharpest nearer to the bone—nerve pain wracking my entire body until it brought me to tears. And I don't shed tears easily.

I live alone and I endured alone—which was fine with me. No way I want to share this with anyone I love, least of all, the girlfriend.

Intense pain lasted until dawn, no matter what I did. I don't tolerate Advil very well, had no Tylenol in the house.

I wasn't prepared. I finally take my temperature later in the morning: 100. Not bad until I remember that my normal temperature has been 97.4 most of my adult life. So, I go into an Urgent Care clinic, see a nice doctor; test negative for flu, and I begin to think that I do have the dreaded virus. But only four people in my town had been diagnosed at that time, and I had been taking precautions: washing my hands often with soap and 91% rubbing alcohol.

The clinic doctor tells me to go home, and stay home; if temperature hits 102, go to ER immediately. Made sense. So, I go home to more pain, coming in greater and lesser waves throughout the day. Second night even worse than first. But too stupid to buy some Tylenol earlier in the day, or maybe I just forgot? Doctors also say the virus can make you stupid. In fact, much of this story is about where my stupidity ends, and medical ignorance begins.

There is no one innocent; we are all complicit. The wretched bastard president did not get elected by accident. And the odd karma is hard to miss: We get this pandemic with this political inanity to boot us in the ass at the same time. I couldn't write this as a fiction—no one would have believed it.

In any event, I will digress so you can learn a little bit about me. I already published eight novels, locally, to good reviews. Went to college; then went to India for a few years to find God; saw enough sorrow and dumb anguish to wonder if there is a God. Then again, I can be a cynical bastard; I grew up in The Bronx. In any event, I know what it's like to be very sick and alone—been there many times in the East of logic.

So, I'm a little cynical and a little stupid and somewhat unprepared—not unlike most of us, even the best of us. Bottom line: I'm just another guy who got sick. My temperature hits 101 the second night, get a rush of chills that cannot be tempered with two down blankets and an electric blanket. And my teeth began to chatter. That was insane, but I tough it out. Pain persists throughout my body in nerve-wracking waves throughout the day—but I tough it again out until my temperature finally hits 102 at 8pm.

On to the ER:

Several things are surprising and hard to believe. I walk into ER waiting room wearing a mask and gloves, and no one is there, not one sickly person but me—never saw that before. I thought it would be mobbed, and especially with people like me.

Two people, who were sitting behind a long, reception desk, invite me to sit down opposite them—I refuse, telling them good chance I have the dreaded virus. They don't believe me. After all, there were only 10 diagnosed cases in my town. And they INSIST I sit down; INSIST I use their electronic pen to sign for treatment.

Then I sit opposite a nurse, further down the long desk, and my temperature hits 102.5. And I get the belated "look" from the two insistent receptionists: Maybe this guy is for real and they insisted on trouble.

Exam room:

I walk a long hallway past many cubicles until settled into a special cubicle. I see a couple of nurses, and a doctor; get chest x-ray (it's clear, and I look up to the ceiling and thank the God I don't necessarily believe in), get poked for 3-4 vials of blood, get swabbed again for flu (negative again), and swabbed for dreaded virus—results in 1 to 5 days: Doc says go home, stay home, wait and hope for the best. But he also tells me I am most likely positive, which I appreciated. Better being truly sick, than delusional. Because that means I'm nuts, which is even more frightening to me than sickness.

Leave exam room after 3 hours:

Three police officers are hanging out in hallway, back far away from me as I enter a long hallway; nurses behind desk who saw me walk down the hallway on the way in, sneak-stare at me as I walk out, thinking: It's *him*. Good chance I am the first person they have seen who (likely) has virus: word apparently spread quickly through ER.

I pass reception desk on the way out. Both "insistent" receptionists are wiping everything down where I sat, then subtly back away and look away: it's *him*. But they meant well—really. Not unlike me, they weren't ready for this dreaded reality. Nevertheless, I was very well treated by all in the hospital within their limitations and my own fears: I mean, who wants to believe this is really happening?

Not me or them.

Best thing for me, and most entertaining came at the very end of my ER visit: It's after 11:00 when I finally exit hospital. There's a guy standing right outside ER doors, likely homeless, ranting and raving about something, and he's surrounded by 5 cops trying to mellow him out. Big electric doors slide open, I slide out of the ER, gloved hands turned upward, and I say, "Guys."

Before I say another word, guy stops the rant, looks at me and walks away; 5 cops look at me and back-off in drill mode: it's *him*. They know it. They can feel it. I can't help but smile behind my mask: Suddenly, I have power; I am special: Nobody is going to fuck with me!

It was first time I smiled in days. I was potent, meaningful. I was special, and I had company for the past 3 hours in the ER.

I was sick, but I wasn't alone anymore.

Nine months have passed, and I'm looking back at what I wrote—and I'm still alone. I guess we all leave the hospital thinking the best, hoping for the best.

And I'm still sickly; at the end of a two-week stretch, recycling covid symptoms, and still listening to doctors on television, telling me how "mysterious" this virus is. And I'm still talking to my doctors, who are likewise mystified because they don't how to treat me, if I can be treated; because I am a part of the first wave, and a lot of what they hear and see in me is new to them.

Least they're honest.

And the wretched bastard president has lost the election and cannot accept his fate. So, he is planning on convening more rallies and parties, and spreading more disease and death. And when reality hits, he will attempt to establish a shadow government under the guise of a political opposition. After all, 70 million people voted for this prick—which is the hardest thing to believe.

Forget about policy; the guy is obviously nuts and these people don't see it? Or they don't care? Or maybe they're also nuts?

It's happened before, in many other countries that went down the toilet—and took millions with them. Like I said in the Preface, in one way or another, we are all suffering this nasty infection.

* * *

It could take us all down, leaving Bill Gates to rein over a world of 200 million survivors in the United States. Which is just one of many wacky conspiracy theories running around America. In fact, I have a few friends who believe in it.

When I asked them how long it would take to kill nearly 8 billion people at the current infection/death rate—if Bill Gates would even be alive to claim his kingdom after they were all dead?

They couldn't find an answer.

And we have the pedophilia ring operating in the basement of that D.C. pizza place—but there is no basement. And the rest of that crazy shit.

Which begs the question: how did so many people go so crazy?

Answer: Greed.

Wanting too much of everything: God, security, freedom, privacy, money, control over a future that can be quite frightening. And wanting it all now; not unlike Trump, whining away in the White House because he didn't get what he wanted.

And, of course, the fear of socialism.

After all, this is the land of the free and home of the brave—like those guys who showed up in the Michigan State House with the fatigues and the long rifles; this is what passes for bravery now; and going without a mask in a crowd and daring a virus to take you down; or daring to believe that the virus doesn't exist.

Tough stuff.

Not unlike assaulting a beachhead in France or a Japanese-held island in the Pacific in WWII.

Not unlike insanity.

Oh, say can't you see
God
Odd as He can be
Creating us no less
More or less
In His own image

Really:
He looks like us?

If that's the best He can do
We are in REAL
trouble

2

This virus can be so weird and sinister, as I discovered. Recovery in itself can be as challenging as the infection—something that is grossly under-reported, or even dismissed by media: Not only can symptoms recycle after testing negative, new symptoms (perhaps originally undetected symptoms) can and do manifest and wreak havoc with mind and body long after having tested "negative."

And there are many indications that this virus can damage the immune system—perhaps permanently. Which is no surprise to me because I am the *infected.* I have been damaged.

And no one talks about the discrimination against the *infected*, being turned away from stores, and having dear friends turn away from me because they are so frightened by what they see on television. After all, I am the infected guy they have seen on TV.

And yet, I didn't want to write about the dreaded virus. In fact, I began working on another novel during the long and complicated healing process, but friends told me I should write about it, and post, if only because I could.

But what sane person wants to relive this?

Answer: when I began to lose my own mind to the dreaded virus; when the challenge of recovery began to rival the sickness of infection; when my sadness turned to a rage against all the inanity and insanity that has manifest in the wake of this weird and sinister virus.

And because I wanted to FIGHT BACK!

I was watching CNN, noting the covid scoreboard on the right of the screen—which tends to disappear when there is even more sensational news: Is this good or bad? I wonder. Right or wrong?

Not sure, but I was reminded of other events that warranted sensational media coverage—like the 2016 election:

BREAKING NEWS: **TRUMP PLANE TAKES OFF!**

BREAKING NEWS: **TRUMP PLANE IS LANDING!**

They gave the wretched bastard enough added/special coverage that they helped elect him to office.

But the media would never admit to that, never admit to their collusion and irresponsibility: not the television news or Facebook or Twitter for that insidious matter.

All jackasses under the guise of friends of freedom—free and dumb enough to play into this deadly psychodrama for another quick buck: as if they don't have enough already.

Greed, as I previously stated—on all sides. The Democrats are not necessarily the good people; they are the lesser of two evils: nearly as greedy, and even as deadly. (Enter Bob Woodward, the legendary newspaper reporter who knew covid was airborne in February 2020, following the Trump interviews, and kept the secret until he published his book in September. He didn't have enough fame and fortune already; he had to let all those people die to attain more fame and fortune. Fucking bastard. And I got sick wearing gloves instead of a mask.)

Meanwhile, the virus eats away at our common sense to work for the common good and save a few hundred-thousand lives and mitigate the sickness of a few million more long-haulers like me.

This virus is so weird; I was getting better yet again and just spent two weeks recycling symptoms: chills, nausea, yellow tongue, muscle and joint pain, rushes of anxiety, extreme fatigue, increased brain fog, decreased emotional control—vulnerable, edgy—another trip to the ER with convulsive stomach pain; this shit just doesn't end. Which is why I ran through the list—for people who haven't been infected, who might be reading this.

You really don't want to get this and see doctors, yet again, who cannot help you, try though might. Because the frustration only adds to the pain.

Having
Texture like black velvet.
But it feels rough
And
Ready to envelope
Me.

Quietly frightening
Silently deadly
All those people dying
Alone.

So bad, so sad
Happiness is
An offense
To this little
Poem.

3

The idea of using poetics to tell this story was unplanned; it just happened, lying in bed at night, unable to sleep and reaching for my cell phone; almost all the poetics were written on my phone—which was completely unimaginable.

Then again, this is such weird story which lends itself to an odd process, I guess. I also thought there would be many more people writing about their own experiences with the virus, who were even sicker than me and much nearer to death; I just suffered an old-fashion, scary ass-kicking: three trips to the ER and two days in the hospital.

Apart from the encouragement of friends and doctors, I suppose I finally decided to write the book out of pure and simple-minded rage. Which is also why this story can no longer be written chronologically, days following dreaded days in linear order of getting it right, if only because I became so enraged, I couldn't think straight all-the-time. Add that to my inability to fight back against so many things gone wrong and unnoticed, and I began to rage—and write.

Big problem is, too many of us are discounting the emotional toll caused by covid-19—just too hung up on the body-count to see what's happening to the *infected,* being killed off by friends and family who won't come near us after—because there is no after—and strangers who even despise us. That is the ages-old story you don't see on TV: about the Mark of Cain this virus has generated.

It took five weeks until a doctor told me I was no longer contagious—which came as a shock because I tested "INDETERMINATE," following two positive tests. Figured I had two more weeks in the house, two more weeks wearing the yellow surgical mask and the gloves—wore the yellow mask for three weeks, the one they gave me during my first ER visit.

Truth is, I loved that mask; it fit perfectly and was perfectly sturdy. And I couldn't find another mask like that, and they wouldn't give me another one—running short back then. And we are still running.

At the end of three weeks, I finally got my hands on a few more masks. But they were nowhere near as good and sturdy and comfortable as the yellow mask. Unless you think I'm totally nuts; remember, humans can get attached to anything, and anyone, and a lot of things that are bad for us.

And I did get into the habit of spraying the mask inside and out with 91% isopropyl, at least three times a day, often enough to delude myself into thinking that I wasn't in the process creating my own special smallpox blanket.

And please remember what I said in the first installment of this story, the dreaded virus can make you stupid. Besides, I only wore the yellow mask about an hour a day (getting the mail in the middle of the night and sneaking a walk around the park at 7am when the weather was nice enough and no one was around after three weeks in the house—because that is also what humans do: take advantage and rationalize.).

In any event, I was reminded of those old westerns, when a band of Indians caught a white guy and threw a smallpox blanket over him to make him feel their pain—probably why I found it so hard to throw the yellow mask away. I was hoping to put it on the wretched bastard president one day and let him feel what I felt.

Out of the house—finally and fit, I thought, after five weeks:

But I wasn't ready for reality; I was so naïve, cooped-up for so long and *SO* self-conscious, despite the doctor's assurance that I was NOT CONTAGIOUS anymore. He explained: The last swab and blood test I took were composed of many markers, and I was negative on all markers except one or two which didn't register anything. Based upon that result and my infectious history, and having had no fever for three weeks, I was NOT CONTAGIOUS. In fact, he recommended my blood donation for convalescent plasma—which still sounds like a thimble-full of a saliva-like substance sitting in a tiny wheelchair. Which might save a life, which is the least we can do.

He also said there was outside chance that there were a few covid cells lurking somewhere in an obscure crease in my body, or maybe sticking to my vocal cords. You see I lost much of my voice during the last week of infection.

ENT Doc said to take lozenges and drink tea if I like, to make me feel better, but that stuff will not heal me; and he had no meds to prescribe for me. And he said there were several possibilities that could have caused the laryngitis: dreaded virus aggravated unknown, pre-existing nodules or polyps, or it directly lodged in my vocal cords. In either case, my voice will likely clear up in 4-8 week—he hoped; he also said expression of the virus could have scarred chords before leaving, leaving me with less of a voice and no choices. At the end of med-call, I asked him what *I can* do:

He told me to pray because he wasn't really sure of what to expect, or what he would find. Or if an errant covid cell could drop down into my lungs.

Which was he didn't want to exam my vocal cords, for fear of dislodging an errant covid cell. In fact, there was a lot of talk of errant cells between doctors. But I am NOT CONTAGIOUS.

And I can donate blood, even if I can't talk very well for a while—or forever, which is truly okay with me considering what I already went through (which I haven't fully explained yet).

Long as I can write, I have a voice. Besides, a musician friend told me I got a great voice to sing blues—like a fucking sledgehammer!

And I am NOT CONTAGIOUS. But no one told me about all the anger and fear I was about to meet when I did leave the house for real to say howdy to the world after five weeks alone with dreaded virus.

Took only three days to discover no one wants to hang out with me, or even come near me for a few minutes, including all my friends who called me and texted me, and emailed me and shopped for me and prayed for me. And I do have a lot of friends, more than most, I guess. Probably saved my sanity, if not my life. And they're not spending too much time with each other either. I knew this, but I didn't *really* know this because I'd been in the house too long, and too wrapped up in the dreaded virus.

I know this is going to sound a little strange, but I'm beginning to think that this may be the most selfish disease I ever had; it took (and still takes) so much out of me, time after time after time; wave after wave of symptoms, and the endless spikes in fever; thinking I am getting better, and not getting better; the trips to the hospital fearing I will never get better; depending on so many others for almost everything because I couldn't do much for myself.

And yet, despite all those remarkable frontline workers putting their lives on the line for us, and dying in the act of saving us, there's some really weird and bad shit out there stinking us up—which is another reason why this disease does not stop taking.

First day out of the house:

I stopped by the hospital to get a pair of gloves on my way home from my first job (I also do color design, and the boys paint the houses, because the books I wrote to such good reviews still don't pay the rent.).

I leave client's house on sunny afternoon, 65 degrees, and I cannot be happier. Was on my way back into town when I realized that I ripped the second white mask, and I was determined to track down a box of those durable yellow masks and share them with friends because too many guys on TV were telling us the virus could last another six months, or even eighteen months.

So, decided I should get the good masks: stopped by the hospital, entered the wide and high lobby (no one in there but me), and asked two reception ladies an odd question: Can you tell me the manufacturer of those yellow masks you are wearing?

They look at me oddly, smile, look at glove box on desk and say, of course. They write down seller's name and address on white post-it-note and slip it under plexi-shield, dividing reality.

To begin with, my hands were trembling: I can't remember the last time I received something in my bare hand from another human being.

Nice lady kept pushing it further forward under plexi-shield, until I finally found the courage to take it. No doubt she could not imagine how self-conscious I was, virtually paranoid. No doubt I was still unaware of how emotionally twisted I truly was: I heard the doctor say I was NOT CONTAGIOUS, but I never "felt" it, was still living it, still walking around the park wearing mask and glove at seven-in-the-morning—not a soul in sight—and still afraid to draw a clean breath and feel the air against my naked hands.

Perhaps the ladies read my distrust and didn't trust me:

In any event, I had planned on shopping at two stores on the way home—another first. And not without gloves. So, I told the ladies I was recently in the hospital with the virus: I was no longer contagious, but still in recovery process, which is why my voice sounded so bad.

They said, "No, it is against hospital policy."

I was stunned; then I asked them for one just one glove and they said no again.

I walked away sullen and bewildered. And then I became really angry. After all the time and effort, I put in, making sure I would not infect anyone else during the last five weeks, these two ladies couldn't help me with one-fucking-glove?

A mask I could understand because they were in short supply, but not the gloves.

ONE-FUCKING-GLOVE!

And I was the only person in the lobby, the only one asking for anything, and I was a real-live virus person—a survivor, I guess—and I am pleading with them for one-fucking-glove with great difficulty because of my quaking, gravelly voice.

I was so angry, so confused; I drove across town and finally pulled over to a curb with tears in my eyes, thinking I wasn't worth one-fucking-glove.

In fact, I cried a lot that day.

I see Earth as Gaia, a living entity.

I see humans as an expression of Gaia, not unlike all else that lives on Earth.

An entity so big and so complex that it often escapes our understanding, let alone our respect; or it may be that we are so deeply enveloped in Gaia, so attached to the Earth that we do not have the requisite distance or perspective to see our destructive part in it, in the body of Gaia.

Regardless, we continue to piss and shit on it. And it doesn't help that the Bible tells us that God created man to reign over Earth—and even to destroy it on a twisted whim. (I am not an atheist; I am a realist who believes much of the Bible speaks to us allegories.)

As if this magnificent, living entity is going to lay down and die for us, for our ignorance and disrespect; it will kill us before we can ever kill it.

Wake up humanity: Anger projected as wildfires; tears expressed as hurricanes; and massive earthquakes and explosive volcanoes on the ever-darkening horizon.

Don't believe me, then keep your eyes on the CNN scoreboard—144,000 covid cases reported today—and tell yourself it isn't happening. And vote for the wretched bastard again in 2024, on the eve of the next catastrophe.

The virus, combining medical, political and cultural issues, has become a spiritual crisis i.e. "The battle for the soul of our nation"—heard that often enough.

In other words, I do not believe that the manifestation of this crisis is accidental. At the very least, it is a timely warning of even worse things to come—from Gaia.

* * *

And maybe you ask why I continue to refer to our (former) president as a wretched bastard:

Because I am sick with recycled covid symptoms as I am writing his book; because I am nauseous, and I want to throw up—yet again; and because so many more people are getting sick and dying and that wretched bastard doesn't give a shit.

* * *

Back to Gaia, who exists on such a deeply complex micro level that we can never see it, and who interacts with other bodies in the macro dimensions of space and time so that we can never imagine it. We know gravity; we cannot even remotely comprehend the intelligent communication between planets or solar systems or galaxies. We measure time in years; Gaia measures it in eons.

I guess astrology is a notable effort at comprehension, or the belief systems of the American Indians and Tibetans; and the Mayans and the Incas who were not so far removed from the life-giving breast of Mother Earth. (A.K.A. Gaia.)

We make no appreciable efforts to connect to Gaia, most likely because we are simply too modern too sophisticated, and too detached, a condition which is greatly enhanced by the advent of technology; I would not say we are too highly evolved. After all, we elected the wretched bastard.

I am also a believer in the intelligence of coincidence: Trump leading us away from healing and loving and caring at a time when it is most desperately needed: Is this just bad luck? Or maybe a bad joke? Or is there a deeper, more penetrating meaning behind this?

Does it matter if the virus came from an open market in China, or from an idiot scientist working on bat-shit in a nefarious Chinese bio-lab, who may have had lunch in that market and spread it to the world?

In either case, humans had their hands on the bat, regardless of their intent; in any event, we suffer the consequences.

WE.

WE fondled the bat.

WE suffer the consequences.

The virus went to my liver, my heart, my stomach, and my voice. And made me cry, yet again.

4

Please forgive occasional reiterations and repetitions occurring in this story, if only because I don't know who will be reading these installments, when or if they will be read in order—and I don't want to spend a long-time editing.

Second day out of the house, I go to local market, a small Whole Foods satellite in my very suburban neighborhood. Hadn't been there in a long time. Went to get ice cream.

Why not? I lost thirteen pounds and could buy all the shit I stopped buying years ago to stay in relatively good shape.

I was walking out of the store when a woman ten feet in back of me says, "Excuse me."

I turn around.

"Are you okay, sir?" she asks.

I'm thinking how she would know I haven't been okay; don't think she knows me, and we are wearing masks.

She is waiting for an answer.

Then I get it. She is waiting anxiously for an answer. She may have been standing behind me online and heard my very raspy voice. "You mean my voice?

She nods.

Shrug and tell her the truth. "From the virus. I had the virus, but I'm no longer contagious."

Her eyes show surprise, relief, fear, and bewilderment—and God only knows what else. In fact, I'm not sure the woman knew what to think or feel; she was so surprised. But I was not at all offended. She was concerned and, most importantly, she was polite.

Twenty minutes later, I went for a curbside pick-up at a nearby paint store and was told to go fuck myself and drop dead, among other bad things, for simply showing up, because two workers there thought I was still *infected*—wouldn't believe me when I told them I was no longer contagious, when they came out to the curb with my order. I was eight feet away—at least.

As they backed into the store, I was about to step forward and pick up my stuff, a move that precipitated the most violent, obscene reaction ever directed at myself. And I took good "care" of these guys at Christmas. And, like I have said, I am a likeable guy.

You see, I was interviewed by the local newspaper when I was sick, because my novels sold well in town. And, as a designer, I selected many colors for a great many houses in the town. Consequently, I know a lot of people.

The newspaper picked up on a few phrases from the interview so, a lot of people knew I was sick, which was the point—and they already knew I was a little weird.

As my health improved, I wanted to help other sick people, especially those who didn't have the remarkable support that I had—even talk to them for a few minutes on the phone if they liked to help them get through it.

We hear the truly dramatic, heartbreaking stories of people who were so loved when they died and will be sorely missed. But we don't hear about the worse tragedies, about the less-loved from smaller families or no families at all—the terribly lonely through no fault of their own, because there is no one to speak for these poor souls. And it isn't good copy.

And you don't hear about people like me—or even you for that matter—recovering from the dreaded virus.

I digress even further to finish this brief installment: After spending all those years in India, studying yoga and meditation half-the-time, and getting into trouble the other half-of-the-time; and after seeing so much sorrow and death, I eventually realized that if I couldn't share what I learned in a meaningful way to help another person, it wasn't worth having, let alone knowing. In fact, it wasn't worth shit.

So, I told those two guys working for the paint store to go fuck themselves.

I had a lot of antibodies, and my infectious disease doctor suggested a lab in a nearby town where I could donate plasma. I got the call from the lab a few weeks later and was concurrently called by a nurse from his office prepping me for the momentous occasion—I wanted to help.

Turned out, it would not be like donating blood: The plasma draw requires a donor, their blood cycled through a machine and then returned to the donor body minus the precious plasma. "Not for the skittish," she said. But I didn't think I would find this difficult.

I was looking forward to it until my doctor called and said this lab was no longer trustworthy, that my precious plasma might wind up in the arm of a wealthy oligarch in Eastern Europe for big money!

Next: another lab in another small town, which was offering as much as $200.00 for a plasma donation; and I was again looking forward to donating, whether I got paid or not—until a friend who worked at the lab sent me a copy of an internal memo: It said that said most of plasma donations from covid patients would wind up being used in an unrelated study—hence the big bucks.

You gotta love America—nothing changes no matter what the challenges, no matter the depth of despair—the fast buck is always first. But I've been in worse places, and I still love this country enough to try and save it from itself—but how?

I'm getting older now and there isn't much I can do except write about it—to a captured audience. Ain't like someone in bum-fuck Idaho is gonna read this and have an epiphany and put on a mask to spare a neighbor's health, or life.

It is all so painful and frustrating on so many levels that this little story can never reach the depths of it, if only because we are still falling and flailing at an ever-escaping dream as we are reaching for the bottom of it.

* * *

I am forced to wonder what the bottom looks like: Is Nazi Germany always the worst-case scenario? Or the fall of the Roman Empire with the barbarians at the gate? Or the dissolution of the Persian Empire? Or the collapse of the Soviet Union?

I think not. After all, this is America: Land of the Free and Home of the Brave so, maybe we simply lose our freedom, very slowly to the point of agony. And we lose our heroism to cowardice—also very slowly, to the point of insanity.

Such a slow and painful death that we won't even know when we're gone.

I wish
I can understand
It
All the shit
That came down because of
It
Not grounded, still floating
Above what's best for me
To see:
Another doctor
Another visit to the ER

What
A way to go
Ass-backwards, in fact
Always no-ing
ourselves
'Cause we don't know enough—yet

5

I learned a long time ago not to listen to a lot of virus news, now down about an hour in the morning, and an hour at night. But can't get too far away. After all, I am writing about the dreaded virus. In one way or another, I remain infected.

I went to Costco this afternoon before the sun came out. And the experience was kind of sad.

I was checking out water pick products in a quiet aisle near front of store. Nothing better than what I already had,

I thought, so I pushed the cart toward the main aisle and ran right into my roommate from college. Hadn't seen him in a while, but he had been very supportive when he found out I was sick; we exchanged a few timely texts, and I was very happy to see him and thank him for support—again.

But he couldn't handle it in person; he began to tremble and backed away in a hurry; he was so scared.

I wasn't offended, but it hurt nonetheless; I would've liked to talk to him a little more.

Back home:

I was listening to woman on the news tell a heart-wrenching story of losing both loving parents to the virus—sounded like wonderful people, so sad. And it played well. The loss of the lonely and poor do not play so well, and there are so many of them, perhaps the majority. And that may be why we are having so much trouble coping with this slow-motion nightmare; it runs deeper than emotion into racial subconscious. It is a PANDEMIC; it is infecting the entire human race. If Carl Jung were alive, he might even qualify it as an archetype. These scars are running much deeper than we dare to imagine.

Later, same day, before sunset:

About 75 degrees and there are so many people in the park near my house, walking, running and riding bikes around the park. And so many families out, more than half the people not wearing masks.

I was stunned, yet again—not understanding what was happening. I hadn't seen anything like this since last summer, let alone the last few weeks, so many people outside.

Just didn't understand, but I had a nice day.

* * *

Gonna write this quickly: Last test for dreaded virus was INDETERMINATE. That was two weeks ago, but doctor said I was NOT CONTAGIOUS. But he ordered another test for me when I told him the difficulty I was having, meeting with so much fear. And I am about to get new test results on-line, at my hospital portal.

Imagine the dreaded virus as a primordial manifestation.

Now imagine the permafrost melting, releasing ancient gases into the atmosphere liberating more ages-old viruses—which begs the question: Can there be a connection between these climate changing events and the primordial fears our president tied into?

Because understanding these people cannot be affected intellectually. Their oddly twisted, Q-induced psychology is not a logical phenomenon; it is instinctual: the racism, the tribalism, the bizarre conspiracy theories. These things are not founded in the brain per se; they are more deeply rooted in our DNA—especially the fear.

It is the dinosaur that lurks in the fog of our souls for confirmation, a fossil of our impotency expressed as fear—like having a tyrannosaurus rex snapping at your ass as you are running through the darkness of your life; you reach for anything to save yourself, become irrational, band together in club-like conspiracies and fight back dumbly.

Against the dreaded virus.

Against science.

Against reality.

Against the future.

Against ourselves in the long run. We keep this up and we will die of exhaustion.

There are nurses working in North Dakota hospitals who have tested positive for covid.

And their own governor doesn't give a shit, let alone our wretched bastard president or the 70-odd-million people who voted for him.

*   *   *

The more I write, the darker this story gets—as if there is no hope.

Of course, there is if we are willing and able to fight back because I believe with all my breaking heart that we must fight back—not from where we want to be, but from where we are; not sometime in the future, but right now or suffer the remarkably indignant and painful consequences.

How many more people must die? How many more people must be maimed?

The future is now.

And good old Joe will not save us by himself, assuming he does take office on January 20th. It will be a relief for a while. We might even see people dancing in the street again on inauguration day; eventually, reality sets in.

Not only Fox news, but Newsmax and OAN (and the Trump Network?) are peddling the same-sick-shit to a waiting audience of those same 70 odd million this time around.

Or maybe you're thinking that one of these promising vaccines will save the day—until the next pandemic, the next season of wildfires and hurricanes. I don't know of one person—regardless their ages or political beliefs—who is not expecting the worst.

This fight; this weirdness; this threat; this fear; these odd people and those primordial conspiracy theories will not disappear for another generation—which is about 20 years, I think.

Until the Chinese grab the high ground on the moon; until we land on Mars.

Until we are looking upward and outward again in the race against implosion.

Negative.

6

Test results: Virus NOT DETECTED!

Seven long weeks to the day since I was symptomatic. I am so happy, so relieved, and so grateful for all the loving kindness and support I did receive. When I write about assholes, or people that are scared into irrationality, they cannot even remotely compare to the good people in my life.

In any event, many of the "good people" still will not come near me—maybe 25 feet at best for a minute or two: they are so scared. And almost all admit, it's the raspy voice they are afraid of, thinking an errant cell could become air-borne following a huge cough that seeps out the side of my mask—even if two doctors recently told me that is HIGHLY unlikely. In fact, I might be the safest guy my friends can meet for a month or two, at least—I hope, depending upon the latest newscast and/or on-line article.

Nevertheless, I have adjusted. I am not insulted. As I said. I made the adjustment after the first week outside. Really did.

Disease:

Looking back on the infection (As if that is truly and clearly possible; as if my mind is clear now.) and comparing to others who were *infected*, I would say I was very sick as opposed to severely ill or critical. And according to the doctors, I was very lucky.

One more bad turn, the virus gets to my lungs, given the intensity of the body/organ attacks, I barely survive, or I die in a few days. You see I head pneumonia twice in one year, not long ago, and I had pneumonia when I was lived in India: I already have enough scar tissue to deal with.

But the infection never took that terrible turn. So, I am another person who "survived" the dreaded virus, for reasons I will never know.

Then again, we are all infected, and we are all a breath away from fate. I learned that from taking care of my mom when she had cancer, when I returned from India: When one person has cancer, the whole family has cancer. Anyone who has dealt with this misfortune will tell you this.

A vaccine by end of this year?

I hope.

But I already know people who will not take it, fearing the motives of the bio-tech industry, let alone the government.

Meanwhile, more dis-ease:

I listened to Bill Maher last week, telling me about eating well and building up our immune systems, making us so durable that we cannot be infected with the dreaded virus. And I agree. This is a good and healthy way to live over time.

The problem is that time is running out. The virus is now, Bill; we are getting sick now and carrots and broccoli won't protect us—NOW.

As much as I like Bill Maher, I am insulted by his detachment—or even entitlement. The guy's starting to sound like he's living in Superman Bizzarro World—

perhaps an adjunct to the Trump World—expressing a version of idiocy and arrogance that belong to the woke-rich-left-of -reality.

Meanwhile, a guy shoots another guy in a Michigan retail store for telling him to wear a mask; many people in Stillwater, Oklahoma threaten violence if they have to wear mask—which is no surprise.

An idiot could have told you: Trump, or even Bill Maher could have told you that this was inevitable.

My concern is that between them, the idiot left and the dumb right, the rest of us may get caught in the ever-painful, irrational squeeze.

It's been eight months since I got sick, and I can safely and sanely say that the virus went to my brain. I am not the same person since I became infected. I can still write and do many other things fairly well. But there are things that I cannot do well anymore, and I have continued to express behavior that is unusual by any measure of my previous life.

I have already been diagnosed with PTSD, and told to get a Brain Spect, which is a low-resolution MRI that highlights brain functions and, of course, dysfunctions. And was also told to get a three-hour neuro-test.

So, I am also a nut job in the making and a candidate for early dementia—if I don't address the issue. Problem is, I am resisting further analysis and treatment because that is yet another indication of PTSD.

Talk about crazy; back to the primordial:

It begins with thunder and the terrifying life of a caveman and/or woman cowering in the depths of their rocky shelter, fearing the wrath of Gaia.

For what? They can hardly imagine, and they began to think about what they might have done wrong to warrant such wrath from the sky—which is the beginning of conspiracy theory: either they did something wrong—or someone else did.

Blaming themselves begets guilt. Placing or projecting the blame outward onto someone or something else begets a conspiracy, which can include a racist thought if you blame someone who appears different than you. Maybe not all the time, but enough of the time to warrant speculation and comparison to our present ugly dilemma.

The foundation of conspiracy theory also has its roots in early storytelling, larger and larger groups begetting greater conspiracies, and a select group seizing power as a result of storytelling, by exaggerating the story to the point of overwhelming the senses, i.e., telling people what they see is not as real as what they are told to see via storytelling, and bolstered by stories about greater powers that lurk beyond the senses. And the wretched bastard president managed to tap into this madness.

And we have ugliness begetting ugliness and stupidity and sickness and the rejection of science and the demeaning of minorities and foreigners.

Sounds like quite a stretch, but unless we are willing to stretch to understand, we will never meet the challenge.

What about tomorrow;
how many tongues lick tomorrow?

7

Nobody I know wants to die today, except the idiot Lieutenant Governor of Texas, who said he would die "to preserve the American way of life." His way of life. But if you are old enough, or poor enough, or dark enough, you'll have a better chance of dying from the dreaded virus in order to preserve the American way of life for the young enough and the rich enough who deserve more of this life.

That's the stats.

I understand being young enough. If this virus or the next is deadly enough, the young must survive at all costs: Fuck the rich—but that will never happen in America.

Because that *is* the American way of life.

I just don't like this wretched bastard president shoving it in my face, having me smell this shit—telling me it's apple pie— before I eat it and die from it. That is insulting.

But what to do?

Interesting how frightened people are, whether it's the virus or the government. And still hard to believe how this president politicized a disease and how many people bought into a fear of socialism—for want of a better word.

I'm not necessarily a fan of socialism, though the ever-widening divide between rich and poor is a concern. And I do believe that all people should have access to decent health care, beginning with a public option at least.

Hard to imagine someone afraid to go to a doctor because they can't afford it.

And interesting how this virus manifest at a time when the health care issue has been a pre-eminent political issue.

Then again, as I said before, I do believe in the intelligence of coincidence: the manifestation of virus, the rise in conspiracy theories, the rejection of science, the bad leadership, the rise in authoritarianism worldwide; it all adds up to something very powerful and most unusual.

Perhaps a change in the pattern of human evolution? Or maybe the last gasp of fear before embracing a remarkable future?

Hard to say, but my experience of these combined phenomena has been a dynamic amalgamation of anger and depression. In fact, nearly everyone I know is sharing in my experience.

And no one knows what to do about it or where it is leading us.

Last doctor I saw told me to resume my life no matter what the difficulties and challenges: work hard, write and exercise no matter how fatigued I am.

So, I am trying to follow his advice. Hence, this book, which is not easy to write, or much fun. Not like a novel, where I can create my own reality and punish the bad people if I like.

In this reality, I get punished each time I turn on the news, or bite into a piece of food I can't taste—still don't have more than 35% of my sense of taste. Thank God I'm not a foody. And I've kept my weight down as a result.

Hard to know, why I feel like I'm floating much of the time; not at all grounded. And the lack of control is also hard to deal with.

And I wonder if this lack of control is also driving these conspiracy theories. Combine that with guilt and we may get some really weird shit projected outward.

* * *

Back to the reality of covid: I saw my PT person today and finally remembered, after eight long months, that it was my call that nearly put her out of business. She had four people working for her back then: five including the receptionist.

Now, she is the only one left working, in an extraordinary effort to keep her business alive.

"If not for your phone call, telling us that you tested positive, it would have been someone else calling with the bad news," she said.

No doubt true, but nonetheless disconcerting that I was the harbinger of hard-times to come—I felt like shit, felt responsible no matter what she said.

And I wonder: Is it a matter of time until we return to normal?

As if the vaccines will be the cure-all?

Far as I can see, we're not that smart anymore.

It was the rage of ages,
and the origin of my silent despair.

8

Meanwhile, I still have people pushing me away—friends no less, they are so scared. And I'm losing my sense of taste again. And I'm losing some hearing, and there is a persistent lack of focus: After 25 years in business, I am making mistakes on bids. Something that never happened before.

And I am missing costly appointments and forgetting to buy stuff in the stores.

And my tongue is turning gray.

And I don't sleep well anymore.

And I don't have energy to keep up with all of this.

And yet, altogether, I am still a lucky guy in many ways, who is simply stressed out in too many ways, which is still better than sitting at home alone fearing the dreaded virus while losing money and my mind.

It was a sunny spring day yesterday. Listening to Eva Cassidy singing Fields of Gold as I drive east of town, passing so many beautiful ranches and farms. Which is a little bit like hearing the voice of God on the road to paradise, the moment is so beautiful.

And then I begin to remember, Eva Cassidy died young from cancer—unrecognized for her remarkable talent.

I'm still thinking about her when I pull up to job site and find my color boards, leaning against the side of the house—trashed. A dozen boards, about 1 by 2 feet each put out of the house under construction (no one living there yet), left to rot overnight in the rain.

My color boards, the ones I made for this job when I was sick and sucked it up between bouts of diarrhea and vomiting, when I was REALLY sick, because I had to make them or risk losing the job (last job for a while I feared). I could hardly imagine the phone ringing with more jobs.

So, I painted these boards under extreme duress, washing my hands with 91% rubbing alcohol, before putting on 2 pairs of medical gloves and 2 masks, so no one else could get sick by handling them. And I kept the job! But I didn't realize how attached I was to those color boards until I saw them trashed.

I just exploded, went totally fucking insane screaming and cursing-inside the house, alone, on a Saturday morning, thinking another trade guy did this for reasons I could not fathom. Because nobody on a jobsite is EVER allowed to touch another guy's stuff without asking—EVER. It is *the* golden rule among tradespeople.

I get so fucking crazy, so blinded by a sudden rush of rage that I call the general contractor—who is a sweet man and a friend. He doesn't answer, so I leave phone message, telling him if he made the mistake with my color boards, he is forgiven because I love the guy; then I go berserk anyway, accusing faceless others who must have done me wrong.

Then he calls me back five minutes later, telling me he has the dreaded virus.

I am shocked and saddened by his accounting of the disease and the uniqueness of his symptoms:

He became so upset by all the bad news about the virus that he began to connect with deeper sadness in his life. He had lost his young son last year, and the sadness caused by the virus finally connected with the deeper sadness from losing his son.

He told me that he spent all day Friday (the day before) crying uncontrollably.

In fact, he was sicker and sadder and crazier with pain than I ever was, if only because the dreaded virus broke his heart.

Idiot's delight.

9

I do like Bill Maher; he can be very funny and insightful.

But, as I said before, I don't always agree with him. In fact, Bill Maher can be an idiot, now comparing the Hong Kong flu in '68 to covid-19 virus, among other stupid shit!

Dumb prick still doesn't understand that it's too late for many of us to get skinny and healthy Which is a great idea if so many of us weren't sick already—duh.

(PS: I was in pretty good shape before the virus got to me.)

Nevertheless, I did learn something from Bill Maher—what an Entitled Democrat is: a human with a dick-in-a-sheep's-ass-backward understanding of the reality for most of us. The idiot is still talking about herd immunity, from the confines of his gated community no doubt, or from the inside of his enormous house—blanketed with security, I imagine.

Would like to see Maher live in my small, two-bedroom apartment for the next year or two.

And then see how he feels about the virus.

Went for a walk around the park, it was sunny, about sixty degrees, and I ran into another old friend on an alley street that borders west side of park. He was driving. I wave to him to stop—haven't seen him in months. He waves out the window after he passes and keeps going. And I know he was going down alley street to park behind his girlfriend's house.

I feel bad, but then he turns around, pulls up to me and rolls down the window and asks how I am.

"You know I was sick for a while?" I ask.

He says, yes, and I tell him I'm okay.

He tells me to back up. I was already six feet away, wearing a mask. So, I back-up two steps and we talk a minute—which was nice. And he leaves me with mixed feelings: He didn't ask me to back up; he ordered me. Then again, he did come back.

Still hurts.

Fucking virus can generate more emotional angst than a passionate love-life gone awry.

I can hardly imagine dying unloved, alone in a non-descript apartment. Or alone in a cold hospital room, one of hundreds of thousands—another number to flash on the evening news scoreboard.

Given a choice, I'd rather sing the blues about a scorned woman who shot me in the belly in a bar one night and see myself dying. begging her forgiveness.

But I was given this reality, and I am doing better with it today.

My voice is improving the last few days—much better today, which is great! But I'm losing my taste again; this infection is so weird. Testing negative does not mean you are symptom free.

More than 250,000 are now dead.

More than 50,000,000 are going hungry.

72,000,000 voted for this wretched bastard and most of them don't care.

We cannot expect them to care. And I'm supposed to find a silver lining in this, according to an evangelical preacher I saw on TV the other night, who was selling heal-all, Holy Water on the side.

I spent nearly four years in India after college, and every teacher I had in India (and in America), which included Hindus, Buddhists and a truly remarkable Christian lady, told me that this crisis was coming, that humanity was closing in on it in a hurry, and that we need to be prepared—to get as conscious as possible, as fast as possible, because there will be an inexorable moment of choice.

Life is not a guarantee, let alone evolution. If the dinosaurs can become extinct, we can follow suit. If one person can commit suicide, an entire race can implode.

For all we know, Gaia may already be planning to replace us with another smart-ass species.

In any event, I imagine that all this speculation is not exactly the stuff of a non-fiction account of a pandemic. But there is nothing else to do at the moment—apart from writing this book and doing color design and walking around the park across the street.

This voidness, greatly exacerbated by the pandemic, must be challenging for a great many people who are tired of all the media coverage—which is distinctly and necessarily negative: Counting bodies and projecting an even greater count of the dead—nearly 400,000 by March 1st.

I have thought of volunteering my free time, but I can't do that much owing to my symptomology, and I can't be placed on a schedule because of the nature of my business.

There are color crises, and a lot of handholding can be required.

And there are very few poor people where I live. In fact, my town is famously wealthy; the whole county is.

In fact, I am an entitled democrat. Middle class for sure, but nonetheless entitled. Some of my doctors actually call me from time to time. I have a Whole Foods satellite store three blocks away from my apartment. I look out the window at pine trees as I am writing this book. And more people are getting sick and dying. And I am not doing anything about it.

This bothers me greatly. I have to do more.

And I turn on the TV, yet again, and I watch the wretched bastard try to nullify an election by compromising the electoral vote in the House. And there isn't a damn thing I can do about it.

This bothers me greatly and I want to do more.

Later in the evening, I tune into Fox news, to the prick, Hannity, and Ingram, the twat, because I want to see what they are scheming, how they are colluding with the wretched bastard. And they have all these guests on, extolling the freedom of Americans to wear masks or not, telling the viewership that most people will do the right thing—as if they had already and the quarter-of-a-million-dead are an accident, if not a fallacy.

I can't do a damn thing about them either. And I wish I could.

* * *

I am overseeing a big job as I write this book, a 10,000 square-foot-house being built for two people no less. And the county is going into a covid, red alert tomorrow—a modified lockdown (making purple the full tilt): closing bars, making masks mandatory almost everywhere in public, telling most of us to stay at home if we can etc.

We have one more day of work inside the house until the floor guys come. But the other workers (carpenters etc.) may not be wearing masks, which is against the virus code red, but in the spirit of the blue-collar mentality—which is how they express their strength and freedom.

What am I supposed to do—rat'em out?

Or go with the flow?

The long-hauler, democrat in me tells me to complain; the worker in me tells me watch my own ass. Which is why I left it up to my guys to work with KN95 masks, which I will supply, or they can stay at home and stay safer.

In other words, I can do something about it, but I won't.

PS: A lot of blue-collar guys I meet on jobs are younger and they want to get the virus and get it over with, thinking they will get some immunity.

And I know a few of them who already became infected and have no regrets. Not sick enough, I guess.

What to say?

What to do, indeed?

Because I'm no better than the next guy, trying to make a living without making waves, without costing anyone else their jobs, or getting anyone sick. So, *we* wear masks and wish for the best.

I am the pain of it,

the life that never
knows the end of it.
Tears not shed
buried behind it.

I am the depth of it,
not to be seen
until the end of it.

10

Recently spoke to a girl-friend who had the dreaded virus and recovered—who still cries every day. At the end of conversation, she finally admitted she hasn't recovered. "I'm just not the same," she said.

All I get is tears welling up in my eyes every day, wishing I could cry, knowing I am also not the same since I got sick. And no one ever talks about the underlying anxiety issues that can come with the virus. And all the other weird and deadly stuff.

Later in the day, I finally remembered someone I knew who had AIDS; a spiritual teacher, no less, who knowingly infected others and killed them.

So, we must understand what's coming—when people like me and this girl-friend-of-mine finally SNAP and likewise intentionally infect others—if it hasn't happened already.

Because that's how some people are.

The longer this virus stays around, the sicker we will become in many ways that are hard to imagine.

And we will continue to devolve, and disinherit ourselves, and delude ourselves. Or else so many of us would not be needlessly crying and dying.

Which can be another description of hell.

This has not been a good day.

This is not a "good" story.

There is a pandemic that may kill half-a-million people in America before it is brought under control.

And we have the wretched bastard president who is attempting a slow-motion coup with the support of sixty million voters who also believe the election was rigged, and a political party that doesn't give-a-shit.

This story is so fucking negative, so redundant with pain and disillusionment, I'm not sure I want to finish it.

After all, it is the madness that makes the motion
And that damned voice in my head
Speaking from beyond the grave
For all those who went
And never returned

11

I've Seen a lot of death in my life:

At last count I made many years ago, I lost more than 20 friends from the old neighborhood to dope before they were thirty. Half of them were close friends and try as I did, I couldn't save them from themselves. And I imagine that the loss of so many loved ones was a part of the reason why I read so much and traveled so much—to find out why and how to cope.

I also saw a lot more death in India—lost more friends there despite my efforts to help them and walked by a lot of dead bodies on the street; then my parents died when I returned home, and I took care of them. And it turned out that people who were dying felt comfortable with me. And so, I wound up taking care of a lot of people who were dying throughout my life. I just knew how to do it. And somehow, they knew I knew.

But I was never successful:

Never saved a life, never overcame my own fear of death. Not even sure how helpful I was.

In a romantic moment, I can imagine myself fighting Yuma, the Hindu god of death—always putting up the good fight, knowing I can only loose in the end.

In reality, I'm just another person trying his or her best to cope and hope for the best, and reel and rage before the dreaded virus returns to kill me or one of my friends.

Fatalistic, Yes.

Effective, unlikely, because nothing seems to help, and no minds on the matter seem to change despite the facts. Which is, yet again, very sad and infuriating, because there is no way to reason with people who believe that the virus is a hoax.

BECAUSE WE ARE NOT LEARNING FROM EACH OTHER AND NOT HEALING. BECAUSE WE ARE NOT MOURNING THE LOSS OF HUNDREDS OF THOUSANDS OF PEOPLE. BECAUSE THERE IS NO ONE TO LEAD US IN MOURNING, LET ALONE RECOVERY. (But I am hopeful; at least Biden got off to a dignified start.)

So much has taken place since I exited reality on this story, including an attempted coup, more than twenty-two million infected, nearly four-hundred-thousand dead.

And a lot of people I know are thinking that this thing might be ending when Biden assumes office.

Really?

I don't think so; I think we are closer to the beginning than the end of the dreaded virus infection and the political instability and the cultural inanity.

The vaccine program has stalled precipitously; not enough people getting vaccinated in a timely manner. And we have about fifty-million people who want a white Christian government, and their faith in this end has not been shaken. In fact, it has been enhanced.

We had Capitol police abandoning their posts, and even enabling the insurrection, taking selfies with the insurrectionists that included former police officers, active military and at least one elected politician.

So, what are looking forward to now: more than a half-million dead, thirty-forty million infected, ten to fifteen million subsequently maimed, walking around like me or much worse than me with bad organs, bad teeth, bad skin, bad thoughts about their futures; bad health insurance if any; another thirty or forty million who will be running around wanting to end our democracy, extolling the virtues of racism under the guise of justice for all.

I never thought I was racist. But I am still surprised to see so many remarkably intelligent black Americans commenting on this fucking mess on TV. Is this surprise an expression of latent racism on my part?

Think it could be, in a very subtle way. I also think that Trump brought a lot of these racist subtleties to the front of my mind. I don't remember seeing a black person and telling myself, "there's a black person," until this wretched prick raised their profile—negatively.

And, as a race, they are suffering so much from this virus and, consequently, require even greater help and understanding.

Meanwhile, I live in a very prosperous suburb, in very white America, and many people in my town are still complaining they don't have enough.

Enough of what?

And those greedy, authoritarian bastards that engorge themselves and control the tech industry, who often vote democratic while they curtail our freedoms for yet another billion dollars—toward what end? How much does one person need?

I'll give you a simple, personal example of how petty and sneaky those tech bastards are: When I publish a book now through Amazon, I am not allowed to have three consecutive blank pages. i.e., they dictate how the content of MY book should look.

I edited an older book cover recently and they wouldn't reprint the book because the cover was *off* by 68/100 of an inch! Yet, they misprint every run of my books by a much greater margin than that.

Next thing they will do is move to edit the actual and sacred content of my books. I have no doubt of that. As a result, and much as I hate to admit it, I do have some sympathy with issues the insurrectionist idiots have raised: There is an appetite for too much control by the rich and powerful. One way or another, we are moving toward an authoritarian future, whether it is fostered by the ultra-right or the extreme left or big tech. And the media. In any event, I don't have a clue on how to prevent this either.

Apart from writing this book, what else can I do? Provide health insurance for my neighbors? Threaten to beat the shit out of Mark Zuckerberg and Jeff Bezos? Drive a truckful of vaccines around the country? Get an AK 47, slip into a pair of fatigues and go to war against those terrorist bastards?

I am so frustrated. And it is so cold and gray outside this morning, and I'm looking forward to yet another day in the house, and another day, and another day. Now I'm convinced it might take another year—at least—until I can walk around without a mask, more likely two years until I can take my ever-present mask out of my pocket.

Yes, I am complaining, and not about the arbitrary intersections of life: shit happens. I had a dear friend who went to a doctor, thinking he had tennis elbow. Turned out, he had a tumor in his lung, pressing on a nerve that went down his arm. Died within a year at age forty-two.

That kind of fate is not what I am talking about, if only because this shit didn't have to happen; we brought it upon ourselves, as I said before.

WE created this mess. WE created the insurrection. WE voted for the wretched bastard. WE created the environment for domestic terror.

WE LOST to Osama Bin Laden.

WE fought the wrong Middle East war at the wrong time.

WE needed to prove that our God is greater.

WE chose faith over fact.

WE denied the reality of Covid.

WE are not the victims of an ill fate.

After all, WE created biological weapons to begin with.

WE are idiots, babe. And it is a wonder that WE still know how to breathe—to paraphrase a great and present poet.

And we're supposed to think that some bat shit got squirted onto a chicken in an open Chinese market, and some jackass ate it?

Maybe.

Or some farm animals were exposed to bat shit and were served in Chinese market?

Maybe.

Or some bio-tech idiot was fucking with the virus in that infamous Wuhan lab, and was inadvertently infected in the god-awful process, and went to lunch, and shit on the rest of us.

Maybe.

In any event, the cause was human error, and the result was catastrophe.

I haven't told you that I have several friends, living in this very beautiful and wealthy, and famously liberal town, who are convinced the infection was intentional; who believe the election was a fraud; who arrived at this conclusion from the far right and from the far left: as if there is a difference between fascism and communism in the applied practice of historical debauchery?

As if this virus isn't connected to history?

As if we don't have barbarians at the gates of reality at another tender moment in history?

As I had said before, I do believe there is an intelligence to these coincidences: How did all the teachers I had—Eastern and Western—see all this coming so many years ago?

How did I "inadvertently" write a sci-fi series about this odd confluence of events fifteen years ago?

How did WE create this fucking mess indeed?

Falling, and
No-body
Looking
Down
At me.
Seeing the sky blue
Close in
On me
Like

Death becomes her:
Who?

It's the
Brain-drain
Speaking
From beneath the reality
Of what happened to me.

12

Like I also said, it took a week of shock to adjust to reality upon healing from the dreaded virus.

But I was wrong: It's been ten months since I was declared negative (on three occasions), and I am still confronted with great fear and huge amounts of ignorance. People are still tightening their masks when they see me, still backing away from me.

And I am still telling myself, "I understand; I understand. I understand. I understand."

Intellectually, I understand.

I am so filled with understanding and compassion that I pulled off the road the other day, into a large, empty parking lot, got out of the car and screamed at the sky like a lunatic?

I'll tell why: Because it's not easy for me to cry. Because each time a person I like backs away from me, it does hurt; it is a form of rejection. And it all adds up to tears I couldn't shed.

So, I screamed at the top of my lungs like a maniac for a minute, got back into my car and went back to my life like nothing happened. But determined to fight back somehow and recover my life.

Or I can spend the remainder of my life screaming at the sky until I lay down and die.

Sunny day today and very pretty; snowed a few inches last night so, all white and wonderful.

I worked for a few hours, then put on the TV and heard news about the House introducing Articles of the 2nd Impeachment. And saw another image of that guy who broke into Capitol wearing an animal skin-type dress, red, white, and blue make-up, and horns on his head, probably thinking he was drawing upon the Boston Tea Party or some other legendary, revolutionary event, for inspiration.

He is likely unaware that the image is iconic, dating back thousands of years to a time when humans emerged from caves and began to gather in tribes, was presented as a wiseman/medium who communed with ethereal spirits, or the Devil himself who threatened all kinds of nasty things, or even the village idiot.

If this guy's a sage, then I'm the fucking Pope.

* * *

Meanwhile, I wound up with a case of trigeminal neuralgia, another residual from covid, causing roaming pain in my teeth and jaw—intense pain sometimes, exacerbated by toothache that drove me insane one night. Next day, the dentist tells me I need seven crowns because I sucked on so many lozenges when I lost my voice for six weeks—which presented several cavities at the gum line.

And my mental/emotional state, though improved, is hardly stable. Got crazy again, got angry at the wrong person because I conflated events. I profoundly apologized the next day, but apology was good enough. Still hurts a lot, and I'm terribly ashamed of myself.

If I haven't told you, the virus went to my brain. And I just have to learn to live with the weirdness and the occasional strange brain, knowing it could be so much worse. And I need to find a creative way to vent and affect changes for the better.

I just don't want to lay down and die.

To that end, I am going to be vaccinated this evening, hoping my mast cell, auto-immune condition doesn't react unkindly to the injection. I was going to wait a few months before I took the first shot, to see how it affected others with my condition, but began to think I couldn't afford to get sick again, while I am still dealing with the residuals of the initial infection.

Yeah, well, next evening:

I'm very sick with headache, chills, body aches, tooth aches, and a 102 temperature. Asked three of my doctors what to expect; that told me not worry. They didn't tell me to expect SEVERE reactions because I am a covid long-hauler, and they are very good doctors and very nice people.

THEY JUST DIDN'T KNOW.

AND WE HAVE A GOVERNMENT THAT DIDN'T KNOW ABOUT THE INSURRECTION.

And the convergence of not knowing hurts greatly and deeply. We are in trouble, people—really deep shit—in so many different ways it's hard to see all the angles and depths.

We're infected in so many ways:

OUR BODIES AND OUR BODY POLITIC.

I go to pieces, she sang
Peace by peace, I hoped
But not so easy pleasing
Myself

What to do indeed?

And there's a fungus among us
No less
Which is a lot more than I bargained
For

'Cept life don't cut that many deals
Which is what the lady was singing about
In the first place when we got fucked.

When we elected the wretched bastard.

And I guess that's why they call it the blues . . .

13

It's a tough time to find wisdom, let alone love and compassion. I've even thought about buying a gun.

In the meantime, I've been watching too much news and so, using my infinite wisdom, I decided to watch *Schindler's List.* Hadn't seen in it in years since it showed on cable. It was so intense that I had to stop watching the movie at least 4-5 times. You see my family name is engraved at the top of Schindler's List:

Dresner—a distant cousin from Eastern Europe, on my father's side, who didn't leave soon enough, from what I understand.

Yet again, the message of the movie struck me hard, as it always had: NEVER AGAIN!

I got so crazy by the end of the movie that I decided to take one of those racist, antisemitic, insurrectionist bastards with me before I die.

Which doesn't jibe with all those Hindu and Buddhist teachings I am familiar with, but does reflect a deep respect for my ancestors and the powerful lessons of history.

The greater sin, under these dire circumstances, would be to do nothing at all and go lamely into the darkness of history.

And pray to the Jewish God that never answers.

I'm also writing in CAPS a lot. Probably because it encapsulates my anger at so many people needlessly dying—now 4,000-a-day. And a democracy crying. And too much time alone.

Tempted to go back to fiction to explain how I feel, but I promised myself I would focus on reality: virus denial, political fraud; lying, cheating, stealing; and an appalling lack of class in the face of a begged favor under duress.

One of the most poignant things that sticks with me is the nine congressmen and women who refused to put on a mask while huddled with others in a small room until the riot danger passed: How selfish can a person be? How callous and disrespectful? How petty and infuriating?

Under the trying circumstances, I would probably put on the mask out of respect for my colleagues even if I didn't share their beliefs.

How deep is the hatred that usurps common decency?

Their hatred, which recapitulates my hatred—which they believe begins with me. But I wouldn't join a crowd to assault the Capitol—even in old days when I intensely disliked the government.

And I would like to stop the virus from infecting and killing other people, even if I didn't like all of them. And I would like to feed all the people on the food lines.

Nevertheless, I had a pretty good day today—until I turned on the TV this evening and listened to Rachel Maddow, telling us that 100,000 people in the United States are expected to die from the dreaded virus in the next three weeks!

100,000 HUMAN BEINGS

The equivalent of filling up the entire Ohio State football stadium on a sunny Saturday afternoon and then killing them.

And I'm supposed to find a silver lining in this?

Meditate for an hour and refresh myself?

Pray to A God I do not understand, who doesn't answer??

Tell myself that things are "bound" to get better?

Or feel the pain and the rage until it moves me to do something relevant and helpful for another human being?

Another thing I did learn from my time in India: Study all you want; meditate as long as you can; learn the Buddhist Sutras and quote from the Bhagavata Gita. But if you can't practice it; if you can't share it with another human being; it ain't worth shit.

It was a bittersweet lesson
In the art of loving myself
Who was without talent

14

I am obviously struggling to understand all this cultural/political madness, without becoming a madman myself; also trying to comprehend the virus in its myriad forms of pain and debasement, if not stay ahead of it—assuming that is at all possible.

I'm trying to remain positive—still.

The first thing I learned about covid is not to buy in, not to think I am healed once and for all, if only because the infection is cyclical. From the very beginning, when I first got the virus, I would feel like I was getting over it every few days, then every few weeks, and now it can be every few months until I express another symptom.

When I think I am over it, that's when I get fucked—or so it seems. As a result, I am trying to take one day at a time, one week at a time—which is a nice way to live anyway.

I am so tired of seeing doctors, and I go through phases with that too—seeing none for a month or more, then seeing three in a week sometimes.

No doubt, it's complicated (which is an understatement); now I'm dealing with higher blood pressure as a result of the virus; it went higher ever since I got sick, and the doctors thought it best to wait before prescribing me with yet another pill.

And I take a lot of supplements with food I can hardly taste—thank God I wasn't a foodie.

No doubt there's a lot to be thankful for: I'm still here, still sound good, still look good (I am told). And still hopeful (but hardly joyous; after all, I remain a cynical bastard from The Bronx. When asked, how are you doing?" no one in my neighborhood ever answered, "Great," for fear the wrathful, Old Testament God would strike them down it they felt too good.)

And no one from my neighborhood thought the government would ever protect them; they were so filled with fear from WWII.

In fact, they often told me that that crazy, German shit could happen here. As my deeply loving mother said, 'Wait, you'll see."

Truth is, she was right about almost everything that was deeply meaningful, my father too.

Then again, I loved being young and dumb. Yet another sad thing is that it must be very hard to experience that state of mind now.

So much for making fun of self-involved millennials who have seen the pandemic, the horror of 9/11, and two economic breakdowns.

* * *

It's another nice day, cold but very sunny, the kind of day that makes me feel lucky to be alive. I'll probably take a walk around the park later. But not before I listen to the morning news, which is a bad habit.

Which yielded ever-sorrowful results. A CNN anchor woman was reading text messages from family members dying from covid—alone, so terribly alone. The anchor woman began to cry as she read the texts and I got tears in my eyes.

Who am I kidding, trying to lighten this story up, thinking it's too depressing: What is too sad? What is not utterly heartbreaking about this? What is not infuriating? What is not shameful?

And nearly half the country is still supporting this wretched bastard?

Where am I living: Land of the free? Home of the brave?

Give me your tired, your poor, huddled masses yearning to breathe free . . .

So, we can kill them with indifference and dysfunction.

It was a dark day
When the change came
In the space between thoughts

When the truth was revealed
And worlds were shattered

15

History does not guarantee democracy, let alone long life and good health. In fact, history demands consistent change for better and worse.

And evolution demands violence. It has been the nature of this reality for billions of years; was the nature of this reality until recently, until Buddha and Moses and Jesus tried to make a difference.

Tried.

I was watching Fox News today, the day of the inauguration; often watch Fox News over the last few months to see what they think, how they think. I usually last 10 minutes until it gets too crazy; sometimes I last longer when I try to project their craziness into my own mind.

Odd, sad thing is they sometimes identify the right problem, like big tech oligarchy, but they always come up with wrong answers.

And I love it when they talk about ANTIFA, who has about 25 members in Portland, 13 more in Seattle and 4 in Berkley. And they rarely talk about the dreaded virus, let alone catastrophic death count. As a long hauler still dealing with this shit, I am offended by the omission; as human being, I find it hard to recognize them as members of the same species.

And I do wonder why Republicans don't seem to get as sick as Democrats:

Because they are rich and protected?

Because they are poor and rustic?

Because they get covid and tell themselves it's measles?

I have heard of people dying from covid who don't believe it. Or maybe I am being as ridiculous as the Fox news anchors.

Another thing: I usually watch CNN or MSNBC and the truth is I'm getting tired of their political slant. I just want the fucking news and can do without incessant analysis—even from the left.

I went to college, read a lot of books, traveled a lot; I ain't stupid--yet. I know a jackass when I see one or a lie when I hear it. I just want the news—without commentary.

Back to virus and the unending, unyielding fatigue I live with, and the emotional imbalance; I am still not grounded. In fact, I had a three-hour neuro test last week for brain fog likely caused by the virus. And I am scheduled for a Brain Spect.

Meanwhile, all my friends talk about is the vaccine; we are all so desperate to return to normal life. But I don't see it; I can't imagine it because I still think we are in for dark times, fighting against our darker instincts. And don't believe the virus is done with me—or us.

I saw a WW II movie the other night and was reduced and shamed by the smallness of my life in view the great sacrifices of so many young people who gave up their lives in that war. As I have said before, we are too self-involved, too introspective—simply too greedy. And too soft.

Now saying the Moderna vaccine is not too effective against the new South Africa and Brazil covid variants. But I'm not surprised; the longer covid is around, the more to worry about—until a strain appears that kills 20% of the infected and QAnon gets more credibility, and Biden becomes incapacitated; and Harris takes over as president, and the madness gets revisited on a scale that dwarfs January 6th. And we eventually get a prick that makes Trump look like a sweetheart.

And we only vaccinate the rich countries, while the poor countries generate more variants.

Not impossible. And if you don't want to believe it, then you are inviting it.

I had a severe reaction to my first dose of Moderna: intense chills, body aches and a temperature that hovered between 101-102 for sixteen hours. But the worst of it is still haunting me, which is severe fatigue after three-and-a-half weeks—can barely get off my bed—and I am dreading getting the second dose in a few days.

I asked two of my doctors if I should go ahead with it, and both encouraged me; both said it was better to get vaccinated and err on the conservative side, because I could hardly stand-up to another virus infection. And they thought there's a good chance that people who already had the dreaded virus with some length and/or intensity may not require a second shot of RNA vaccines. But no one will know for sure until more data is gathered.

Meanwhile, the Congressional idiots gave Taylor-Greene 199 of their precious votes to remain empowered; quite a pair, the Q-queen and the wretched bastard, who pass for heroes no less, and it's still hard to imagine what kind of odd karma this country is answering for—apart from systemic greed and racism.

And yet, bad as this country can be, it is still better than most. I still want to believe that; I began to believe that when I returned from my long stint in India after college. I was happy to come home and was grateful to remain. Problem is I ain't living in the same (sane) country anymore.

Are you?

Odd thing is many people on the right feel the same way and accuse democrats of taking away their freedoms. And they are very good at it—until you hear the one about not wearing masks under any circumstances. i.e., I can get you sick if I want and you can get me sick, and we can maim and kill each other.

I keep coming back to this argument if only because it so clearly demonstrates their perversion of freedom—and Christianity: Am I my brother's keeper?

Obviously not.

* * *

And now "nap" apnea, yet another covid symptom which recently appeared during my seemingly endless nap time every day, me waking up gasping for air—this fucking virus is so weird and sinister.

Do trees grieve
The loss of leaves
And reflect upon
The dead reds and yellows and browns
And turn green with envy in spring?

Does life and death rhyme
In the mind
Of God only knows that the devil
is in the details of how sick and
crazy we really are?

16

Another nice day today, cold but sunny. Another good day to be alive—even with the pain and tightness in my chest, which is, hopefully, a physiological defect and not heart related.

Is it covid-19 related?

Who the fuck knows; I've experienced so many symptoms since contracting the disease. And I've been tempted to list them all, but ultimately pass on the idea because I always imagine how depressing that would be.

Then again, I'll give you my "favorite": yellow tongue.

Had thrush when I first got sick, a white tongue, followed by two expressions of yellow tongue. And no one knows why, and everyone tells me not to worry.

I just google with some prescribed solution and brush my tongue, and it goes away in a week or so. And returns a few months later.

Seems harmless to the point of ridiculousness, which is why I 'like" it—because I can conquer it; I can control it. Then again, I am forced to wonder if it is a sign of a weakening immune system, something not so easily corrected.

Interesting how people want to believe that we are returning to normal when we reach that mythological goal of herd immunity.,

WE ARE NOT RETURNING TO NORMAL after 6-700,000 dead and 8-10 million maimed by persistent side-effects: after the assault on the Capitol and more—a lot more.

This "thing" is so complex, so insidious, so challenging that it's gonna take someone a lot smarter than me to figure it out.

Again, I refer to the convergence of significant events: the virus, the politics, climate change etc. And I repeat that instinct tells me the simultaneous arrival of these events is not accidental; these are life-changing, world-changing phenomenon—sponsored by evolutionary necessity to adapt or disappear.

The problem is: I can't even deal with simple one-to-one relationships, which are derived from this crisis. I mentioned this before, but I now believe it is worth going into detail.

I left the house one day, about a month ago—another nice sunny day; was walking to my car thinking good thoughts, when a dear lady friend drives by, slows down and parks.

Exits her car with a warm smile and asks how I am doing etc. I hadn't seen her in a while. After a virtual hug and exchange of pleasantries, she starts telling me about the "fraudulent" election.

I tell her, "Gimme a fucking break, seven million votes across thousands of counties, involving tens of thousands of voting machines . . ."

She hurries back to her car and returns with pages of "facts" to back her claim.

I took a cursory look and said, "It is nice to see you," and did my best to avoid confrontation.

Then I drive to the job site, and run into another friend on the job, who casually refers to the election fraud, and I casually move onto a more pressing job-related subject.

Then I come home and get a call from a very close girlfriend, a devout, evangelical Christian with a heart of gold—this is a woman who practices what she preaches; this is also a woman who long-believed that elite Democrats engage in pedophilia and drink the blood of children.

But we don't talk about the election—purposely—if only because we silently agreed to disagree about many related things following the debacle at Charlottesville.

And then the insurrection at the Capitol, with people wearing labeled, antisemitic t-shirts: Camp Auschwitz and 6MNE (6 Million Not Enough).

We haven't spoken since, probably because we both don't care to address the issue of me telling her that she is, inadvertently, supporting rabid ant-Semitism.

She doesn't believe it because she loves me and many other Jewish friends; she won't believe it until the day "they" come to ask her where Robert Dresner lives, and she will not only tell them my address, but will drive them to my house—to protect the lives of her own family.

What the fuck am I supposed to about this: Back further off and never call these friends again, and let the love die on the poisoned vine? Or argue the point yet again to no avail? Or even tell them to get fucked and why?

A big reason why I didn't want to write about this issue is because I believe in Jewish-prudence: not unlike many other Jews, I don't want to engage, am even embarrassed to engage; do not want to shout too loudly that "I AM a Jew"—if only because that is how many of us were raised with my mother telling me, "Down deep they don't like us. You'll see," when I was still young enough and idealistic enough to embrace the world and think better of it.

Again, please know that I am not a religious Jew, though I was Bar Mitzvahed. And I have studied a bit of Kabbalah, and I wrote a novel about the Jewish people. Though not religious, I have always identified myself culturally as a Jew—and proudly.

And now more so than ever, and not unlike Muslims who became more devout when they felt their lifestyle threatened by the West, and the Christians who reacted to show their "greater" faith.

And now me, the Jew, who is going to affix a Mezuza to his door—which I suppose is a timely gift—to display and enhance my identity.

What to do if another pickup truck parks in front of my favorite coffee shop this summer (it's happened before), with a front license plate denoting a convoluted Nazi symbol: Say nothing? Do Nothing?

And go silently into to that coming night and the next day and the next day and hope it all turns out okay because this is America—after all?

Really?

It's the
Oddity
Not the sadness or the badness

I'm not the only one losing
Touch
I ask people
All kinds of people
And they say it's the madness

And yet it's all somehow familiar
Me—not unlike the people
I wrote about who went to Mars
Who felt like they had been there before

too: Et tu Brute

17

The wretched bastard ripped the scab off our prejudices at the pitch-perfect time to reveal the endemic weaknesses in America—during an epidemic.

It also revealed to me the power of precedent. I had no idea, until this mess started, how much of our country was founded on good manners and common sense passed from one administration to another, a much-heralded process, which has lasted for hundreds of years.

I had no idea how fragile our institutions are—how one guy can wreak so much damage to them in a few years.

I also thought that we had the ability to blunt a pandemic with relative ease. I thought we were much smarter than that already; and was likewise unaware of just how powerful the Internet was, how much negativity and hatred and frustration prevailed in America and how deftly it was connected and usurped by political interests.

I was asleep.

I could not imagine feeling so sickly eleven months after I contracted the virus. I missed the first half of the Superbowl (which was a terrible game in any event) because I was so fatigued, I could not sit up on a couch and focus on the TV.

So, the doctor told me this morning to cancel my second Moderna injection and wait a few weeks for more data to be collected on vaccines for long-haulers.

In the meantime, covid restrictions have been modified in my county; restaurants are allowed 40% capacity.

Really? When every doctor on TV, and almost every medical article I read online tells us to beware of the new variants, how quickly they spread.

Saw another doctor yesterday, discussed latest symptoms that include chest pain—yet another symptom that started two weeks ago. So, he ordered an echocardiogram and a nuclear stress test; then saw another doctor today who ordered thyroid ultra-sound and blood work.

It doesn't fucking end!

It doesn't fucking end!

But what am I supposed to do—nothing, and wait for the end?

Got the TV on in the background, was listening to Fox news—for the usual ten minutes, until it got too fucking crazy—then switched to CNN and heard Carl Bernstein refer to Trump an evil man.

I agree.

But I can't do anything about it, and that particular frustration visits me every single day—my utter paralysis. And this journal I'm writing isn't going to help very much; I expect that I'll wind up communing with a sympathetic audience.

I still don't think I'm going to change anyone's mind. As I said before, I have trouble speaking to some of my dearest friends about the Q nonsense.

What to do indeed?

As I understand it, there were about 160 Capitol police fighting off the insurrection, and I still wonder why they didn't shoot any of the rioters—in the legs or in the ass at least, especially if they thought they were protecting people's lives inside?

I mean, fuck these people.

Then I wondered if Capitol police carry guns. So, I googled it and couldn't get a straight answer. I've noticed that a lot lately, getting harder and harder to get simple answers to straight questions on the Internet; a lot of ads and a lot of other bullshit meant to distract the user.

And that is how people seize and maintain power in America now, in business and politics: by obviation. The more these entities maintain your attention, the more you are likely to spend, or even believe.

In one form or another, you are required to surrender yourself; you are bartered and battered to surrender yourself.

It ain't only to the wretched bastard: it is the surrender to products and politics and conspiracies. And we now have a whole generation that was born to surrender, and to malign and rat-out friends and families—anonymously.

Yes, the COVID-19 virus is an oddly, organic mirror into our digital devolution of thinking and feeling—and eventually our breathing.

Think about it.

Hint: negative replication; mass vaccination:
Think
There is a history of
Coincidences
And/or
Accidents
That alter the course of
Recapitulation and Evolution

Until history takes a second look,
And realizes that
WE
Are no accident:

Dinosaurs had to die
For us . . .

Ever wonder what we have to do?
If we have to die to make way for the next leap in evolution?

18

Or are we already doing it to ourselves?

Maybe the biggest problem with Q is the faithful thinks too small.

In the meantime, I continue to feel like shit—I am severely fatigued—and I keep on hearing how the vaccines may not work very well—if at all—against the South Africa variant. And I still have to decide whether I should get a second Moderna shot, which may suck me dry and leave me housebound.

And the longer I have less energy, the scarier it is. And all of a sudden, I am having problems with my morning prayers and meditation; can't seem to focus.

No, I don't pray to God, as if He has time for me among several billion galaxies—or even universes—being born and dying; I just pray for people hurting as a way to connect with their sadness and challenges. And I sit for 20-30 minutes, which isn't very long, but suddenly too much—since I got the first Moderna shot.

Now I'm one of more than forty-five million who got vaccinated, but I don't hear stories about people like me, whose reaction was so long-lasting from the first shot—8 weeks! Still reading same-old medical articles online.

I've been writing this off and on for nearly a year, always telling myself to make sure everything I write is somehow related to the dreaded virus, always wondering: what isn't?

Another one of my friends lost a child. They found his frozen body floating in a lake. He was suffering from traumatic brain injury; as a result, struggling against drug addiction for a long time. A good kid with bad karma.

No matter the cause, the pain for his mom is nonetheless the same for too many moms and dads I know. Add a pandemic to that horrific sorrow—the inability to have a normal funeral or memorial, the compounded grief—and you also begin to wonder how the dreaded virus impacted this kid's life and tragic death; it could not have been helpful.

In fact, every breath we take, every thought we have, everything we feel is virus-infected—as I had said at the beginning of this account, and nothing has happened to change my mind.

In fact, I am afraid the vaccine might even affect our perception of reality going forward: how quickly we can be moved to forget and continue to facilitate the next dreaded virus by intruding upon nature yet again, building ever-deeper into our forests and jungles getting ever-closer to a horrific end rather than a new beginning, if only because we are too fucking stupid and greedy.

In any event, I have a decision to make; I have heard that there is a memorial planned for the kid who lost his life. And I must decide whether I should attend or not? Mingle or not? Attend and stand back? Or not attend and send a note?

I have also begun to wonder whether I should tell people that I am still sickly because some people are still afraid of me, still thinking that an expression of covid symptoms implies contagiousness.

And I wonder if I haven't been too negative, perhaps too cynical in my assessment of our futures since the onset of the pandemic.

Of course, I can see things working out in the long run. After all, we have survived two world wars, a civil war and a depression, and more: why not survive this crisis intact—or even improved?

I can imagine improvement—until I turn on the TV and hear about the censures issued to the few Republicans who voted to impeach, how the far right, lock-step conformity to the wretched bastard persists; how forty percent of the electorate bought the big lie, that Trump won the election by a landslide.

And I hear from a doctor espousing a belief that we are already nearing herd immunity; and another doctor fervently disagreeing with him.

And I see how I am feeling this morning, like I should go back to sleep because I can barely stand up—and I wonder how my own covid difficulties might be affecting my own point of view?

And I am about to confront one of my republican friends about their beliefs in elite, democratic pedophilia et el, wondering if it's even worth effort—yet again?

Because I like her so much and I don't want to lose her friendship—by supporting system that is bolstered by white supremacy and anti-Semitism.

I still don't get the systematic beliefs, why so many people who believe in one righteous thing (i.e., being against abortion) have to believe in all the crazy shit that has been attached to the entitled "woke": the pedophilia, drinking the blood of children, and the massive attack on our sanity by the implementation of a 5G cell phone network, and the Jews using space-rays to ignite wildfires.

No doubt I ascribe most of this crazy shit to the right, if only because they are already nuts. What if the left follows suit to defend itself and it gets crazier?

It's not impossible.

In fact, it's probable in one form or another—if this thing, this crisis, this craziness proceeds unmitigated, or unchallenged, if only because it will not go away like so many of us are hoping.

What if I postulate—bluntly this time, adding no poetics to what I really think—that maybe a return to normal is wistful at best?

I already said, in so many ways, that we are all infected.

What if I told you that WE are the variant, and that there is no return, that our evolutionary pattern or thrust has already been altered by the much-dreaded virus and that we are just playing out our roles in an odd sort of fate?

If you think I'm nuts,

Think about Q.

It's night
Time
TV on-golf:

Recorded white noise.
Looking up at the ceiling
Fan
Unmoved for last 6 cold months

Switched to news
Switched back to recycled golf
Eyes back on ceiling fan
stuck on

Duh-pression

19

I don't think about Q very much, don't have to. All I need to do is to look at myself: I might get healthier, become more energetic, but I will not be returning to normal in this life.

I know this in my heart and in the depths of my soul.

I have also read *The Mind Parasites* by Colin Wilson and never forgot it: the story was simply genius, suggesting that an alien intelligence can somehow traverse space and time, in the form of parasites, and enter our minds organically—we just inhale them.

I won't go that far, characterizing covid-19 as alien; like I said, I'm not that nuts yet. But I can go as far as I see in the changes taking place in the human psyche right in front of me.

This is not 1918. This is the future; we are talking about the Moderna and Pfizer vaccines affecting our RNA in ways that are similar to digital intelligence.

I just heard it again on the news, yet another doctor gushing about the miracle of the vaccines—which may be true—then comparing these creations to the machinations of digitalized thinking.

It is also true: when we begin to change our RNA, we begin to change ourselves in ways that are presently unfathomable. WE ARE entering the world of sci-fi as I write this journal. WE ARE already living in the era of "double-speak."

That wretched bastard, former president was no accident; in fact, he was predictable.

I was sitting on the front porch of a new friend a couple of years ago, a brilliant woman and a world-famous athlete. And the conversation became quite intense and most interesting when it turned to the advent of Trump—who she referred to as "the joker.'

This kind of errant force that shows up from time-to-time, in the human evolutionary scale, to remind us that we are all-to-human, if not crazy stupid.

And we have survived them all, thus far, and moved on—to what? And to where?

We landed on the moon more than fifty-years ago and spent the subsequent time finding new ways to implode, looking inward instead of outward; looking at each other for satisfaction and exploitation and not at other possibilities beyond us.

In fact, we are cannibals of a sort, eating our own hearts out.

We are not reaching.

We are taking and gouging and getting fat-headed to the point of this journal recording the experiences of another sick person who is sick and tired of being sick.

Yet another fucking doctor: I was so happy today when someone cancelled an appointment and I got to take their place—much earlier than I was previously scheduled. And that made me happy—THAT!

I was so busy being born
And dying
And so sick sometimes
I didn't know whose life I was living.

20

It can be embarrassing to be so angry and small-minded. In fact, I am tempted to delete some of the stuff I've written (especially the craziness about getting a gun). I can hardly imagine how many people in this world wished they had my access to medical care.

But then the reader wouldn't know what it's like to have the virus, to still have the virus, and be driven to utter exhaustion for nearly six weeks following the first Moderna shot.

Then again, we have Texas suddenly steeped in a deep-freeze—and unprepared to meet the challenge of climate change. And we have a mayor of a town in Texas exhorting the survival of the fittest: the weakest be damned and dead; the government not necessarily responsive or responsible for anyone's lives.

This guy is like Sam Houston and Davy Crockett rolled into one brain-freeze, imagining he is living in the wild frontier with a population of 20,000 in 1836, and every man, woman, and child for themselves—free to kill or be killed.

And I think I'm nuts?

Rush Limbaugh is dead, another sweetheart. Died from cancer; should've died from the virus he derided. Fuck these people.

I'm sitting at the back of a large wait room, waiting for an echocardiogram, my mind wandering and wondering. Saw my first doctor this morning and tried to "reason" out my predicament with his help.

Because we couldn't (which was not surprising to either of us), he asked if I would consider upping my Cymbalta to a therapeutic dose, thinking my depression may be the result of severe fatigue.

I said, yes.

Why not? Yoga don't help, meditation don't help. And he has made some helpful suggestions before. I have gotten better--until the inevitable worse comes calling. Meanwhile, I don't think I have a heart issue, but can't afford to guess wrong so, I will take this echo-test and the stress test tomorrow. And another test and another test until I won't do it anymore cause I'm better, dead, or just sick and tired of being sick and tired.

Still amazes me that I found the energy to write this little book.

Then again, maybe not because I could have written much more, much faster if I wasn't dealing with viral symptoms.

So, blame it all on the virus; it is easy to do, it has been at times. But how much blame can you place on an illness?

Somethings, if not most things we are born with—in our DNA or maybe from a past life: take your choice; in any event, we are all born with predispositions.

After all, I was an occasional suicide as a kid, which was another reason why I went to India, to find out why I was so sad. Was it Karma?

No trip to India, and there would have been no life left for me; I am convinced of that. Which is also why I wrote so many books, to rationalize my life, to lend it meaning and share that attempt with others looking for something similar.

I am still looking—still living, and perhaps the one implies the other.

I go in for echo-test, and lovely lady test person and I begin to talk.

She asks: What am I am being tested for.

I tell her covid related chest pain--maybe.

She's very interested because she contracted the dreaded virus in November—not too badly—but scary enough because she lost a cousin to virus complications, which ended in lethal meningitis.

She's better now but "not the same person," she said. She just doesn't "feel" the same." And she still clears her throat regularly. And I was reminded of the all the people I know who had the virus and tell me the same thing. "I am not the same person. I just don't feel the same."

Like an all-too familiar mantra.

In fact, WE, the infected, are not the same as we were; will not be the same: how many times, how many ways does it have to be said?

How many millions of us have to repeat it until someone can make sense of it all?

I had pericarditis, hepatitis twice, bacillary infection, amebic dysentery twice, Mast Cell Activation Disorder and more, and after all that, I still feel like the same person; and I still managed to recover much of my life; I almost died 3 times from a variety things and circumstances, had a gun put to my head in the middle of the night, in the middle of the desert in Afghanistan, and I still felt the same afterward—if not a little lucky.

And this fucking virus makes me feel different?
Like I'm someone else?
What don't I understand?
What am I missing here?

What if this virus is alienating us from ourselves?
What if that is a genuine side-effect?

The second doctor I met today was a revelation—I hope. I recently heard about a primary care doctor in town who was treating covid long-haulers so, I made an appointment, figuring what do I have to lose?

The guy had an excellent reputation.

Turns out the doctor was not focused on virus people, but on patients with chronic and/or complicated conditions; he had only seen five covid cases before me. So, I was a bit disheartened; ten minutes after he began to speak with me, I was enthralled.

Not only was this doctor a sweetheart; he was brilliant. His specialty was neuropathways, a relatively new science of healing, which sounded more like a form of Zen meditation, how our brain neuropathways are turned off and on by pain; how it is our brain that is experiencing pain and not our body; and how previous experience with pain grooves the memory of discomfort and becomes hyperactive, poised to see pain or generate pain from the mere thought of it or the fear of it.

And how these neuropathways act similarly with emotional pain. This doctor was not offering me a cure or another pill; he was raising the possibility of symptomatic relief through mind alteration, a change in point of view on a subtle level of awareness.

Leaving his office, I thought this approach can be helpful, and I began to think about all the help I had already received and all the kindness that has been shown to me by so many medical workers during the past year—especially the nurses and the receptionists (which is a long way from not providing me with a cheap rubber glove in early May).

Based on their kindnesses alone, I should learn to be more grateful.

And more enraptured by the miracle of life expressed through the eyes of one exceptional receptionist; eyes so blue, yet so green; so bright and vibrant—hazel electric might be the best way to describe them.

And she always wears a black mask, which always focuses my tired eyes on hers, and makes me believe: Yes, there is a God burning brightly within us.

It also made me wonder if am not a misogynist because I can't see past her eyes?

And it made me realize that this country is so fucking crazy it wants to nullify magic.

"What kind of man is he?" she asked.
"Like any other man, only more so," Bogey said.

I wanted to be more,
But I'll take what I got,
It could have been so much worse.

21

It's another sunny, winter, Saturday morning—quite beautiful. And I'm hoping to walk around the park today, and maybe meet a few friends at a local coffee shop (outside and socially distanced).

Amazing how much I've been missing these little social gatherings: coffee lunch, an occasional dinner, how much of my day-to-day life was defined and supported by these gatherings; so many of us miss this routine—all over the world, I imagine. In fact, can't imagine a trip to India that wouldn't include much time spent in a local chai shop.

Most amazing was watching the animated footage of the Perseverance rover landing on Mars and seeing the first magical pictures of the Martian landscape. After all, I did write a five-part series beginning with the first manned mission to Mars. I did stretch my mind to write those books.

I wanted to live long enough to see that species-defining endeavor take place in my lifetime. As I've said before, I want to look out and up, and to stop looking at my fellow beings as political enemies or carriers of a deadly virus. I continue to be struck by the convergence of events that has pitted us against each other; more so now than ever. And as Biden says, it may not be until next Christmas before we can welcome each other with a hug.

If we're lucky.

I still don't get a good feeling about all this, as if there is still more to play out—medically and politically, more to suffer in dumb anguish, grasping for straws of understanding and extended moments of relief.

People who say, "one day at a time," are wrong, maybe dead wrong. If there has been anytime in my adult life to provide for a secure future for the species, it is now.

It's a sunny Sunday morning. I had a good day yesterday, until 3:00, when I had to lay down and nap until dinner. Nevertheless, something did come up in the evening, which I may have to deal with next week. If it's a nice day next Saturday, I'll meet a few people for coffee again—outside. And two dear old friends, who have been particularly scared of the virus, plan to show up for coffee for the first time in a year.

If they are afraid to sit near me, I will smile to hide my hurt and anger. I'm just so tired of this shit, so concerned I may have to get an anti-body test to back up the vaccine shot just to walk around with it to put someone else at ease—like I did last May when I lost my voice and walked around with a negative test in my pocket to "prove" I wasn't contagious.

Maybe you're thinking I'm a weird guy with weird friends (especially after reading this account of my life).

No, not the case, looking back on the year. There's 10-15% of people in this town that are careful to the point of paranoia. Though I understand the situation, I can't say I like it. I can't say that I will continue to indulge it much longer, telling myself how much I understand it, and that it's okay.

Because I need to get better and if I can feel better walking away from them, fuck them and I'll walk and watch out for my own emotional welfare.

And I am forced to wonder how many other covid people have to deal with this; I don't really know because the subject matter is greatly under-reported.

Meanwhile, I'm the guy who said I'd wear a mask just to make someone else comfortable if they were afraid of the virus and I wasn't.

Is there a difference between that and walking around with the results of an antibody test (and vaccine shot) in my pocket?

Then again, who wants to think about this shit?

I am hopeful that the science of neuropathways will help with all of this: being all too human to the point of petty stupidity.

No doubt, this book is filled with all kinds of mixed messages, and emotional turmoil, and a few hypocritical, self-righteous statements. And in that respect, it may well be compared with some of the far-right, Q bullshit.

Difference is, I know I'm a little nuts.

And I'm trying to get better.

I want to be "normal."

I saw a third doctor this week, the cardiologist who encouraged me to write this book. Another sweet man, and also very bright.

He assessed my cardio-related test results and said, "You look beautiful inside."

Which made me smile; he also thought my chest pain could be derived from issues with my digestive track—if not another covid conundrum.

I left his office feeling much better, perhaps energized, but ran out of energy by 2 pm. This doctor also told me to give in and take rest when I get tired, and to maximize my output when I had energy—which made sense.

Problem is, he told me not to give in to my fatigue when I saw him three months ago.

But it's not a problem because his understanding of the virus has changed since then. Not only has he encountered more patients like me, his cousin, a doctor in another state, has been in the hospital for the past two months with the virus, fighting for her life.

I woke this morning wondering if I'm petty to the point of narcissism, being so concerned for my welfare, seeing all these doctors, taking all those tests when there are so many more people out there much sicker than me. And some things have improved lately; nap apnea is suddenly gone, and I got 7 new crowns, and the trigeminal neuralgia is better. (At least I could afford the crowns by having the boys paint the dentist's house, and I cannot help but wonder about the many people who cannot afford this.)

In any event, it all comes in waves, the expression of new symptoms, the recycling of old symptoms, and the doctor visits and the medical testing—every couple of months it seems—and now it's the reaction to the Moderna shot.

What to do?

What to do indeed?

Yet, it still feels indulgent.

But in some odd ways, I'm sicker now than I was a year ago—because of that fucking vaccine shot—just when I was feeling better, I had to do that to myself and suck out my life energy.

And make myself more crazy; and then write about it and make myself self-conscious to the point of embarrassment because I don't want to appear weak and slovenly; thinking I'm better, wanting to be better, but feeling worse. And afraid to admit it to people.

But it's still better than dying from the next variant, so I should be happy I took the first shot despite the complications because it is yet another sunny, winter morning, and when I walk outside, I'm gonna breathe clean, fresh air and have better thoughts and greater hope.

* * *

8 FUCKING WEEKS on my back because of the first vaccine shot—no fucking energy. Out of the house at 9AM if I have to be, home by 11 or 12, and back in bed on back until 7AM the next morning—for 2 fucking months!

They should have tested me for antibodies BEFORE I got the first shot.

And there is no fucking anyone is reporting about people like me on TV, because it would help ruin the vaccine program—which I hope with all my heart is for the greater good.

In any event, you don't watch out for your own ass, you can and will loose it.

Bottom line:
I was just so hurt and lonely.
sometimes,
I just wanted
someone to touch me where
it hurt the most.

22

I've had the virus for a year already, so long it seems like I've always had the virus—like I don't know myself without having the virus. And people out there (doctors, politicians) are still telling me that there is a return to normal.

Hardly. I am damaged goods: The so-called long-haul ends when I end.

I AM NOT MYSELF.

I AM NOT GOUNDED.

AND I REMAIN DEEPLY DISCONNECTED.

And I wonder when this "issue" will be addressed that we, who are known as long-haulers, do not "feel" the same anymore: what is the root of this odd feeling?

Is it solely biological, the result of an odd infection?

Is it symptomatic of the disease compounded by social/psyche issues that have permeated the society for the past year?

Is it something else?

Or are we afraid to think outside the box of idiocy on Facebook?

If there is anyone left in America who still thinks that this is just a virus, they are just fucking stupid.

As if the wretched bastard was a quirk of politics?

As if QAnan is an accident of history?

As if I will ever come to terms with my Q friends?

Fuck do I know; some of them prayed for me and shopped for me when I was sick.

And some of them are anti-Sematic by association. And racist by ignorance. And authoritarian by way of self-righteousness.

Meanwhile, my energy level has improved greatly during this past week—seven weeks after my first Moderna shot. And my stomach is better, and my chest pain has noticeably diminished.

Am I, in fact, healing?

As if I haven't asked that question a dozen times before.

* * *

I just got the results for my Brain Spect: evidence of trauma and infection throughout my brain; doctor believes it is mostly infection, likely derived from covid. Lab Tech analysis of images suggests issues with anxiety and mood dysfunction. Which jives with my expression of edginess and vulnerability, and profound disconnection since I became infected.

Doctor also believes much of it can be mitigated with the use of infrared therapy—so, I remain hopeful.

And curious, having just read a medical article wherein 30% of all people sickly with covid-19 have sought psyco-traumatic analysis to explain their issues with covid: Why didn't their doctors order Brain Spects?

Why are these people settling for less?

Why does this pressing aspect of covid go under-reported?

* * *

I often wonder how I would have related to the virus if I was much younger, in college maybe: Would I be respectful of the virus in its myriad, horrific expressions? How often would I wear a mask? Would I be especially careful in the process of dating? Would I stay home a lot more? Spend a lot less time with the boys?

Yes and no, knowing me, who could rationalize almost anything when I was in my early twenties. In fact, I knew everything worth knowing about life when I was in my thirties—and I loved knowing and swaggering around like I knew it all, and I would love to do it again.

In the meantime, at this point in my life, I don't know shit—which is what my parents told me would happen. In fact, virtually everything they told me about life was true.

I might have said this before, but it is worth repeating, reminding myself that I had a lovely family growing up.

It's a cold and snowy day. I'm looking out the window as the flakes fall on a tall evergreen tree, listening to yet another TV doctor in the background, telling us we have a good chance to return to the new "normal" yet again—by the end of summer this time.

Fucking idiot: Is it normal for hundreds of thousands of kids to go on spring break with wearing masks when a pandemic is still raging?

Is it normal for states to suspend healthy protocols BEFORE many more of us are vaccinated?

Is it normal for us to wear a mask from time to time, have an occasional dinner inside a restaurant with dear friends and family, carry an ID card validating our vaccine status (and subtly questioning other people's vaccine status in the way people questioned my health status—I already know people who are lying about their vaccine status)? Is it normal to figure how much fencing and barbed wire would be necessary to secure the Capitol, how many National Guard troops need to be stationed nearby? Is it normal to defend our political leadership against assassination on the job and even in their homes? Is it normal to wait for the next variant, the next booster shot, the next pandemic? Is it normal to wait on the next climate change catastrophe?

Is endless, fucking greed for everything under the sun normal?

Excuse me: I mean the "new normal," which includes a credible attempt at mass voter suppression with the intent to elect a white supremacist autocracy.

I'll tell you what I think normal is—the bottom, fucking line: when this society ascribes to living by the compassion expressed in THE SERMON ON THE MOUNT and honors the sentiments etched in bronze on THE STATUE OF LIBERTY.

When health care is available to all in need; when all the mass casualties are behind us; when people learn to give as much as they take from each other and from nature; when they can apprehend the miracle of life and its preciousness;

when we can meet our destiny in the stars; and when we greet each other in peace.

When things get so bad
and so sad,
and we beg the dusk for dawn.

And drop to our knees in awe and in thanks,
when we can finally
see clearly
nearly every drop of sunshine
emanating from behind that
long and lazy cloud
straddling the endless horizon.

Lest we forget, we are the variant.

Author's Note

I did my best to convey what it's like to be sick with the virus for a year. No doubt, there are many redundancies and contradictions throughout my story. And there are several things I am still inclined to delete—as I have said before, if only because I don't like the idea of appearing weak or indulgent, or neurotic or petty—let alone crazed.

Not unlike everyone else, I want to look good to the world. But there is nothing good about a pandemic and the other weird shit that has accompanied this sinister infection—unless, of course, in some ass-backwards way, we learn something immensely important from this debacle, which is how to survive ourselves, if not flourish.

Stay safe, be well,
Robert

* Special thanks to Dr. Nelson Trujillo, Arsen Kaskashian, Orion Black and Schwartz-Neil for their unerring support and encouragement.

** I live in Boulder, Colorado, where ten people were massacred inside a grocery store, and no one can tell me that this horror isn't yet another expression of a greater affliction that is morphing us and killing us.

Covid-19 is not only a disease; it is a symptom.

So much has changed
Looking different
Feeling different

We are not the same
Too many maimed
And dead

Thinking otherwise is
Not seeing
Who
And
What we are not

Again and again and again and again
Against all reason

To behold the future-stillborn
Made of cans
And sand

If we only had
more sense
To lose our heads
And make a gift
Of our wishful being
To the master of the moment

Which is: $\mathbf{E = mc^2}$

POSTSCRIPT (November 2021)

In layman's terms, when applied to the current human condition, the relativity theory looks like this: At the height of an impending crises, there must be a certain quality of collective awareness present in the human race to surmount the crises or it faces extinction.

In the old days, this was explained as the coming of a new avatar—when the world reached a critical imbalance of good and evil, Christ was manifest, Buddha, self-realized etc.

Now, it may be up to the entire human race to bind together and save itself: WE are the Avatar. And I can't say we're looking too good at this moment in time, but I remain hopeful or else I wouldn't be writing about it.

Also, I can't remember when I first heard about this application of the relativity theory. I think it came from reading the Alexandria Quartet, a four-book fiction by Lawrence Durrell set in Egypt during WWII. He based the entire tetralogy on the theory of relativity.

Even if the application I recalled isn't exactly true, it sets the tone for this journal: we don't rise to this singular occasion, we kill ourselves. In the meantime, people still ask how I feel, and I tell them, "Pretty good lately. At least I don't feel sick anymore—just tired sometimes."

Which is not entirely true. I just don't complain that much anymore, and I learned to accept the vicious cycle of symptomatic recurrence—which is now measured in weeks—not in days anymore. Which is good.

And I remain a bit brain dead because of the virus, but I am learning to live with that too. (I passed on infra-red therapy because I didn't like the trauma shrink that authorized it, and because several other doctors believed that the Brain Spect only showed a moment in time and may not be a log-term indicator of the problem. I will eventually take another Brain Spect, and if it matches the scarred etchings of the first, I will likely get the infra-red treatment.)

The biggest and longest lasting covid issue I am dealing with is this odd kind of detachment, a curious lack of grounding, a subtle anxiety that is almost physiological. And the accompanying sense of vulnerability, which is still coming at me in waves that can be quite disconcerting. Fact is, I am not the same person as I said on the back cover of the book.

And I suspect that these symptoms are not unique to me. In other words, we may have 20 million people previously infected by the dreaded virus walking around like zombies—fatigued and ungrounded.

But much of this stuff remains under-reported because the continued spread of covid-19 by the unvaccinated is the sensationalized headline news occupying this magicless moment. And the need for a booster, which I will not take upon consulting with four doctors: one urged me to take it and risk another extreme reaction; one was uncertain; two doctors said it wasn't worth the risk (after testing 2500 H on a Total Spike test and 20.00 H on an IGG). Which were encouraging numbers, if not debatable.

Turns out the quantity of antibodies are no longer as important as their quality. But there is no test for quality covid-19 antibodies.

In any event, I remain heartbroken by the events in Afghanistan. I spent nearly a month there many years ago, traveling overland from Herat to Kandahar to Kabul. It was the most remarkably primitive place I had ever seen and, consequently, enchanting to a young man wanting to learn about life the hard way.

And now what? We leave an entire generation of free and educated young women bound to the violent and repressive Taliban? And we say we're so sorry to their family members who worked for us, that they are not our responsibility. Then we shouldn't have educated them and used them to further our own self-interests to begin with. We shouldn't have lied them and deceived ourselves.

Which should not come as a big surprise from a government that can't handle a virus—among other things. Where are the accurate, rapid test kits? Why does the messaging continue to be so unclear? Why are the vaccine mandates so hard to implement? Why is the Democratic congress so dysfunctional? I thought Biden was better than this.

I thought WE were better than this. As a result of the virus, people who were already sick became sicker; people who were already nuts got crazier; people who were not nuts and angry became fearful, generating conspiracies manifesting in selfishness, under the guise of righteousness in a misguided effort to unravel a democracy.

Once again, I thought wrong.

POSTSCRIPT

We are broken, my friends. In so many ways, it is hard to calculate, and it is getting harder for me to identify with any political party.

And it is getting hard to believe that the dreaded virus will leave us any time soon. Not unlike the flu, I am afraid it is here to stay with us and define us for many years to come, along with those selfish bastards who think it is their right to choose what is good for their own bodies (with some mindful/medical exceptions) no matter what the infect is on other bodies they share their pitiful lives with.

My rights, my body, my freedom—MY, MY, MY: My God, it is a wonder we don't die from (self) consumption.

And yet I am still hoping for the best, still waiting for that special challenge that will bind us with caring.

PPS: And now we have the promise of pills, and a doctor on TV telling us that the pandemic will be over in a few months: Really?

Perhaps they may even develop a remedy for selfishness one day, and I am forced to wonder how many people would take that pill?

Made in the USA
Monee, IL
08 November 2026

67378676R00073